How to [barcode] a Puppy

The Beginner's Guide to Training a Puppy with Dog Training Basics. Includes Potty Training for Puppy and The Art of Raising a Puppy with Positive Puppy Training

Brandon White

Text Copyright © Brandon White
All rights reserved. No part of this guide may be reproduced in any form without permission in writing from the publisher except in the case of brief quotations embodied in critical articles or reviews.

Legal & Disclaimer

The information contained in this book and its contents is not designed to replace or take the place of any form of medical or professional advice; and is not meant to replace the need for independent medical, financial, legal or other professional advice or services, as may be required. The content and information in this book, has been provided for educational and entertainment purposes only. The content and information contained in this book has been compiled from sources deemed reliable, and it is accurate to the best of the Author's knowledge, information and belief. However, the Author cannot guarantee its accuracy and validity and cannot be held liable for any errors and/or omissions. Further, changes are periodically made to this book as and when needed. Where appropriate and/or necessary, you must consult a professional (including but not limited to your doctor, attorney, financial advisor or such other professional advisor) before using any of the suggested remedies, techniques, or information in this book.

Upon using the contents and information contained in this book, you agree to hold harmless the Author from and against any damages, costs, and expenses, including any legal fees potentially resulting from the application of any of the information provided by this book. This disclaimer applies to any loss, damages or injury caused by the use and application, whether directly or indirectly, of any advice or information presented, whether for breach of contract, tort, negligence, personal injury, criminal intent, or under any other cause of action.

You agree to accept all risks of using the information presented inside this book.

You agree that by continuing to read this book, where appropriate and/or necessary, you shall consult a professional (including but not limited to your doctor, attorney, or financial advisor or such other advisor as needed) before using any of the suggested remedies, techniques, or information in this book.

Table of Contents

Introduction 8

Chapter 1: Puppy Training For Beginners 15

Chapter 2: General Tips and Info Before Training Your Puppy 19

Chapter 3: Techniques And Tips To Train Your Puppy 24

Chapter 4: Potty Training for Puppies 26

Chapter 5: What Breed Of Dog Will Be The Best Fit For You? 29

Factors To Consider 30

Chapter 6: Physical and Mental Exercises for Your Dog 37

Chapter 7: Understanding Dog Psychology and How Their Minds Work... 46

But First, How Did Modern Dogs Come About? 46

The Psychology Of Today's Modern Dog Breeds 47

Understanding Dog Pack Hierarchy and Why It Matters 49

Building Boundaries 50

Chapter 8: Choosing Your Pup's Bathroom Location 59

Chapter 9: Correcting Behavior Problems............ 63

Shushing the Barker 64

Barking for Attention 64

Barking at Everything... 65

Not Accepting Biting 67

Getting Chewing Under Control............................. 69

Stopping the Digging Frenzy 70

Discouraging the Jumper 72

Chapter 10: Methods of Housebreaking.............. 74

Paper Training... 74

Crate Training.. 76

Litter Pan Training 79

Crazy Training Plan 81

Chapter 11: Top Techniques to Train your Dog 84

Make use of his paws.. 84

Jump.. 85

Teach him how to leap 85

Act like a Man 86

Spinning Around 86

Jump through hoops... 86

Roll Over 87

X Marks the Spot.. 88

Shake it off 88

Chapter 12: Secrets of Living in Harmony with your Dog 90

Open a Door...90

Let us Count! 90

Hush, Hush..91

Fetch...92

Jump Rope..92

Keeping his toys 93

Chapter 13: Other Important House Training Tips 94

Chapter 14: Dog Treating 97

Chapter 15: Dog Nutrition....................................101

Raw Food Stuff..103

Chapter 16: The Beginning of a Good Routine 105

Water and housebreaking 107

Chapter 17: Guideline on Puppy training............ 108

Reward 108

Tone.. 110

Positivity 111

The Perfect Pro to Train Your Dog 113

Chapter 18: Dealing with Separation Anxiety 115

Conclusion 119

Introduction

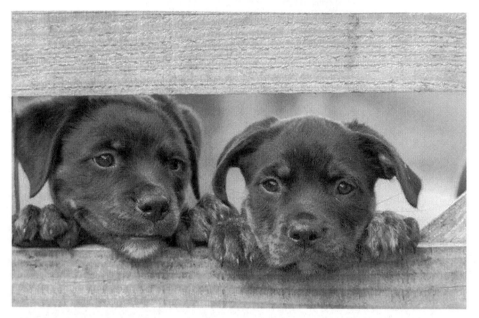

Every species, human or not, have to go through a period of training. If you think about it, humans have one of the longest training periods of any species because it takes us years to learn how to talk, walk, run, jump, and learn the millions of facts we are taught in school. As young children, we repeat many of the things we are learning to cement them to memory. Our parents are consistent, patient, and considerate in teaching us about morals, ethics, values, safety, and all the other things we have to learn.

So why would it be different for a young puppy, a few weeks old? Your puppy has to go through a learning process. The more consistent, patient, and consideration you show your puppy, the easier it will be for him/her to learn what is expected of him.

As puppy owners, we can forget these concepts. We can forget, in our busy lives, what it truly took for us to learn all that we did to become intelligent, responsible adults.

It might be easier for you to learn how to train your puppy, by thinking along the lines of how long it took you as a child to be obedient and well behaved. It is why numerous puppy training books often mention over and over that you need to be considerate, consistent, and patient with your puppy. Now that you have been reminded, you can go on to learn the truly important aspects of training.

Animal behaviorists study the psychology (behaviors) of animals, such as dogs. Through their work, we have a better understanding of puppy behavior. Your puppy lacks vocal cords. While, he/she can make sounds, he/she is unable to tell you how they feel, what they want, and it is your job to read their behavior. You also need to understand the character traits, and tendencies your puppy breed is known for.

Puppy Psychology

Puppies are infants that will grow at a quick rate. They will be born with certain instincts and then it is your job to teach your puppy what he/she needs to know. The puppy's mother uses imprinting, such as requesting the puppy to sniff a smell and providing a stimulus to show whether that smell is good or bad. You can do the same. Imitation is fairly easy to understand. If you bark, your dog will bark.

If you turn off the TV at night, call your puppy, and go to bed soon you will find all you have to do is turn off the TV and go to bed. Your puppy will learn that the TV off at night means bed. Through habituation, your puppy knows the routine.

Associative learning is a process where you introduce a stimulus and request a new response. Pavlov's dogs are an example of associative learning. He taught dogs to salivate to a noise versus food. At first, he would introduce meat powder into the controlled environment with the dogs. Soon the dogs started salivating before the meat powder was distributed. He then took the meat powder and a ringing bell, where he predicted the dogs would soon start to salivate when the bell rang, without meat powder being distributed. He was correct. The bell became a neutral stimulus and the meat powder was the unconditioned stimulus. The study aimed to show that a stimulus would elicit a response from the dog and that one could train a certain behavior. Most of what your dog learns will be through associative learning because you will provide a stimulus, ask for a certain response, and reward your puppy.

To train your puppy, you will need to provide a motivational reason or reward. Puppies are motivated by their instincts to have food, water, shelter, and love. Your puppy is going to want to have action in their lives. They will also have needs and desires.

Your goal is to meet the needs, desires, and teach appropriate actions, while ignoring the inappropriate behavior. Consider a toddler for a moment. A toddler will learn that negative responses from you get them attention. For example, if they throw a toy on the ground when you are talking and you pick it up, the child will throw the toy again if they want you to pay attention to them.

Puppies will do the same thing. They can develop negative behaviors simply because you provided a response to it. Even a "no" is better than being ignored in a puppy's mind.

Your puppy has emotions. They can be sad, happy, depressed, bored, worried, or fearful. A puppy's vocalizations and body language are two ways you can determine what your puppy is feeling. Their actions are another. A protective puppy will stand in front of you and defend you. A confused puppy may lay his/her ears back, tilt their head, and look at you with those soulful eyes.

Stages of Puppyhood

Puppies need their mothers from 0 to 2 weeks. During weeks 2 to 4, there is a transitional period, where the puppy is starting to eat puppy food versus milk, and they are eventually able to leave their mother and be with their owner. Between 4 and 12 weeks is the socialization period of your puppy, where he/she needs to meet other dogs, people, and learn how to interact. If you have other pets in the home, 3 to 6 months is going to be a ranking period. It is a time where your puppy will learn its position in the household. If your puppy has a dominant personality, he/she will try to establish their alpha ranking. Puppies are adolescence starting about 6 months to 18 months. Depending on the breed, your puppy can reach adulthood at one or two years.

Character Traits

Your puppies' character or personality traits will start to develop at seven weeks. Their full personality will be evident by 10 to 12 weeks. To choose the right puppy, it is best to wait for week 7. Start to visit your puppy and at week 10 to 12 evaluate your puppy's personality again. The environment your puppy is in will also determine the character traits you see. Your dog may act completely different in their home turf versus in a new home.

Genetics is going to factor in with regards to personality. Since this is not a book listing all dog breeds and traits, it is in your best interest to get a book on the dog breeds you are most interested in and learn about their genetic predispositions.

Non-genetic character traits are something you will need to observe. These traits will develop based on your care, love, and how you meet their needs. A puppy can also have different personality traits around different people because they understand what is or is not acceptable.

For instance, a dog might go to work with its owner for several months. The dog is then left at home with another person. The new person ignores the dog, works, and provides a stable play routine. The dog learns to sleep, play on their own, and ask to go to the bathroom. However, when the dog goes back to work, he doesn't associate this same behavior. Instead, he is rambunctious, gets into everything and demands attention. It is because the owner is now seen as a play partner. The owner comes home and plays with the dog, so now the dog thinks play time is whenever the owner is with him. He/she starts to show that he/she isn't going to listen because he/she wants to play. He/she tries to assert dominance over the owner to get what he/she wants.

Tendencies

Tendencies are typical puppy behaviors seen in breeds. For example, scent hounds have medium energy levels; they are easily distracted, and are very social animals. As you read about your puppy's breed, you will find a list of certain tendencies, which will help you determine how to train your puppy.

Cool Facts:

- Approximately five to 30 minutes after your puppy eats, your puppy will need to go to the bathroom, most often defecating.

- For each month of age, your puppy can hold their bladder approximately one hour. This means an eight-month old puppy should be able to hold his/her bladder for eight hours.

- Goldsmiths College, located in London, has shown that dogs feel empathy for owners and strangers.

- The University of Vienna determined dogs understand when they are being mistreated.

- Dogs have more olfactory receptors than humans, thus they have a heightened sense of smell, which you can use in training.

- Max Planck taught a Border collie 200 vocabulary words. It shows your dog can learn words, their names, and commands through proper training.

14

Chapter 1: Puppy Training For Beginners

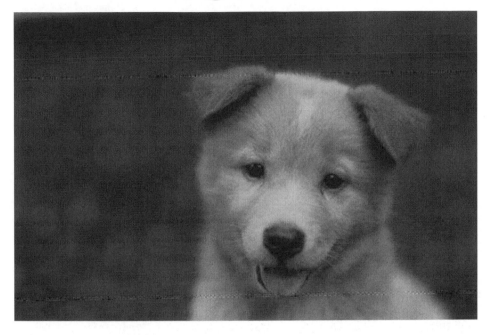

Puppy training can start as soon as your dog enters his new home. In fact, the way you receive the puppy is already a training-starting period, allowing you to set the tone to what is about to come.

One thing to keep in mind is that dogs take their cue from their owners. Hence, the way you behave will affect how the pups behave. This is why quality breeders make a point of asking about a buyer's emotional and financial ability in taking in a new puppy in their home. That being said, here are some of the things you should keep in mind when preparing to be a first-time trainer of your little pooch:

Safety First

Once puppies are weaned from their moms, they stop being protected by their mom's immune system. Hence, there's a strong need to start vaccinations and de-worming ASAP to ensure that the pooch is protected from common health problems like parvo. Make sure to ask your seller for the pup's vaccination records so that you can continue with the process. Routine visits to the vet for injections may continue for the next 3 to 4 months of the pup's life.

Puppy Diet and Schedule

Most new owners don't realize this, but puppies can have a hard time adjusting from one diet to another without proper introduction of new food items. If you're bringing home a puppy from the breeder/pet shop/adoption agency, make sure to ask the people in charge about the pup's diet and daily routine. Inquire about the food they feed the pooch and purchase the same brand from the store. If you intend to change the puppy's food brand, you can do so slowly by adding a little bit of the new food to the old one. Being aware of the pup's original diet and schedule lets you build up on this information and change it to fit your own lifestyle. You'll be amazed at how the pup's diet and routine can help with the training program.

Dedicate Time

Puppies take time as they start getting used to their new surroundings. You might find yourself waking up in the middle of the night to the puppy's cry or having to clean up some "accidents" in the living room floor. Sure, you'll be able to teach the pup toilet training pretty soon, but that doesn't mean you are completely safe from having to wipe urine off the carpet. That being said, make sure you have enough time to set aside for the puppy, preferably getting one during vacation or extended leave. Like babies, having a puppy usually means going home directly after office hours to keep the little fur ball company.

Patience is Crucial

Your dog wouldn't immediately learn how to sit, stay, or even how to tell you if they need to go to the bathroom. Hence, it's important to hold on to your patience. Some training may require at least a week of teaching before the pup manages to pick it up, and he's bound to forget what you've taught from time to time!

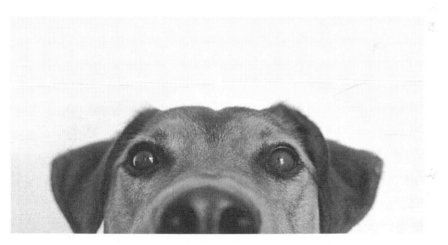

It's a Family Effort

If you live alone, consistency in teaching your new pup shouldn't be a problem. If you live with others however, it's important that your teaching and behavior methods are basically the same. For example, you might determine that letting the pup on the bed is a bad habit, but your significant other may have a different idea.

It's best to talk about these things beforehand, especially if you have children in the household. This way, the pup doesn't get confused about what the humans want them to do.

Know Your Breed

Breed plays an important role in puppy training. Some breeds learn faster while others require a more stringent approach for training. Later on in this book, we'll talk about the most common dog breeds and how to best address their training. In the meantime, go online and check the profile of the pup you intend to have. This should include characteristics, energy level, grooming requirements, friendliness with kids/pets, and more.

Chapter 2: General Tips and Info Before Training Your Puppy

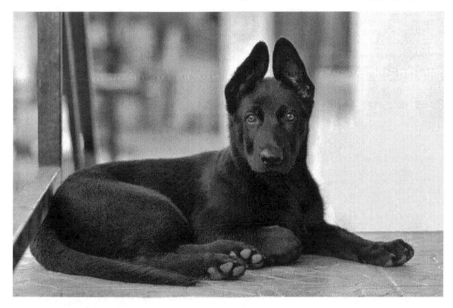

What would happen in your working life, if you provided a report one time with no errors, but the next time there were errors and you continued to have an inconsistent pattern? How did you learn how to type on a keyboard with accuracy? As a child, when you were instructed to do something, such as "please, clear the table" and you didn't do it, what happened? What happens when someone asks you to do something, but you don't understand their words because the phone bleeped out? How do you feel when you get reprimanded versus rewarded at work?

- For inconsistency, you probably get retraining and told that after a certain period of time, without improvement you will lose your job.

- Learning to type you had to repeatedly practice.

- If you did not do as asked, you were disciplined, and requested to follow the request.

- If a statement is unclear, you ask the person to repeat and then follow the request.

- When you are given rewards, you feel 100% better than when you are reprimanded. You might also feel embarrassed due to the reprimand or feel it was unjustified.

The best tip that can be offered to you—is to think about your puppy like you do other humans. Your puppy has emotions, but needs time to learn. You are given chances to be consistent, repeat, and follow requests. Your dog has to be given the same consideration.

Consistency

To obtain consistency from your puppy, you must first be disciplined enough to provide the same consistency. If you work for one hour on the sit command and then go three weeks before you work for another hour on the same command, your dog will have forgotten everything they learned the first time. Providing a routine for your puppy is how they learn.

It is not just about training commands, toileting, and other aspects. Consistency is about the routine you provide for your puppy. Each day you get up at a certain time, your puppy gets up with you. What happens during that day?

Sample Routine:

1. Your puppy gets up

2. You let your puppy relieve himself/herself because it was a long night of sleeping

3. You feed your puppy at the same time each day

4. You prepare for work, and your puppy prepares for the day alone or perhaps with you

5. You come home, let your puppy out, give him/her lunch

6. You go back to work, and your puppy goes back to their daily routine of being alone

7. After work, you come home to let your puppy out, feed him/her

8. After your dinner, it is time for puppy play

Of course, somewhere in your busy daily routine, you have to train. Your puppy is going to listen better if he/she is not fully energized after a boring day. You do not want your puppy tired either, but you do want some of the energy to be run or played out.

Make sure you are consistent with the routine and training each day.

Repetition

Repetition is not only done through consistency, but also in those training periods. You got your dog to sit after giving him/her a treat. Now, you will repeat the process. On the third attempt, you ask your dog to sit, but give him a different type of reward.

If your dog is not listening to the request or does not understand you, repeat the voice command once. Guide your puppy to show them the behavior you want. Ask your puppy for the behavior. When your puppy provides that behavior, give a reward, and repeat the command, until your puppy is no longer confused.

Voice Commands

A common mistake among dog owners and voice commands is too many words. Your dog can understand one word and associate it with a behavior. Through repetition, you can give one command, praise, and follow it with a second command, such as sit and stay.

First your puppy has to learn to sit. After sit is known and always followed, then you can start training stay. Eventually, your puppy can learn a string of commands, but always start with simple, one word commands.

Rewarding

Rewards need to vary. If you give your dog a treat every time they follow a voice command, you are simply teaching your puppy that for the stimulus they need to provide a response and it will always be food. If they do not get food, then they will refuse the command. By rubbing down your puppy, saying well, or giving a treat, your puppy learns that he/she gets something it wants, but it will not always be food.

For example, if your puppy jumps up and down at the door, you can tell your puppy to sit. When the puppy sits and stays, then you open the door and reward them with what they already wanted.

You're Mindset

Your mindset is just as important. If you lack patience you will have a tendency to yell, threaten, or physically punish your puppy. All of these are horrible because your puppy just lacks training and understanding. You are your puppy's parent. You are responsible for keeping your emotional control and the appropriate patience.

If you cannot, then sit quietly. Be calm in your body language and facial expressions. Wait for your inner self to calm down, and start over. Your puppy can read your body language and facial expressions, just as much as the tone of your voice.

Have you ever noticed a dog tuck his tail and lay his ears back, when someone yells, but is not yelling at the dog? It is a natural instinct to tuck in, and feel empathy for another person.

As long as you can remember that your puppy is like a child and that consistency, patience, voice commands, repetition, and rewards all help you train him/her, you will succeed.

Chapter 3: Techniques And Tips To Train Your Puppy

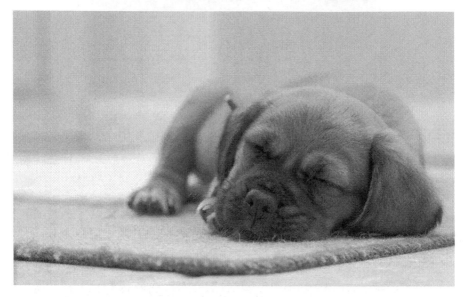

Puppy training often requires some hacks, tools, and tricks to make sure that the pooch pays attention and remembers what you're trying to teach. You'll be surprised at what factors can actually affect the pup's ability to learn! That being said, here are some factors that you should keep in mind while teaching.

Exercise Is Important

Exercise is something you should definitely introduce to the puppy on a daily basis. Like toddlers, puppies have a very large capacity for fun and play, making them very energetic. Unless all this energy is burned off, there's no way the puppy would pay attention to your training strategy. This is why it's best to start training after the pooch has enjoyed a good run, allowing them to become more compliant with your teachings.

Time Your Teachings

Timing refers to the optimum time when your puppy is most receptive to teachings. Obviously, you'll have to teach the pooch after exercise, but repeating the lesson several times each day would prove more effective, allowing the pooch to easily remember the command. The best time would be when the pooch is compliant, not overly tired but still has sufficient energy to listen to what you have to say. Mid-morning and afternoon would be perfect since the pup should be spent energy-wise during these times. Note that lessons should be kept short but repetitive throughout the day. Twenty to thirty minutes of your time for every lesson would be perfect since puppies grow bored easily and are unlikely to remain attentive after 30 minutes.

Use Tools

The use of tools would make it easier for you to achieve the results you want. We're not talking about electric shock collars or anything like that, however! For most dogs, a collar, leash, clicker, and treats would be enough. A crate is also crucial when it comes to toilet training. For more elaborate techniques, you can try buying some hula hoops, tubes, and others – but only after the pooch has learned all the basics.

Chapter 4: Potty Training for Puppies

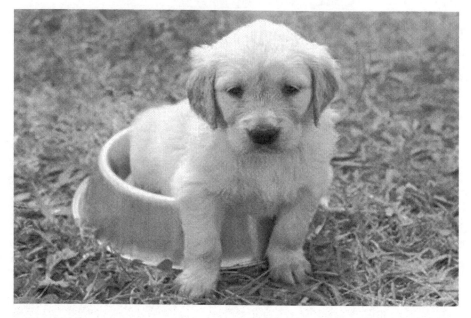

Like babies, puppies have very little bladder control so don't be surprised if you encounter "accidents" during the first few weeks or even moths of the pup's life. In this Chapter, we'll talk about the different things you can do to speed up the toilet training process.

Designated Pre-Toilet Trained Area

It's usually best to keep the pooch contained in a single room of the house while he hasn't mastered toilet training yet. This will keep you from finding wet puddles and poop all over the house. The kitchen would be the best place – just install some baby fencing to prevent the pup from wandering around. His food, water and bedding should be kept in one corner of the kitchen, preferably somewhere easily seen as you enter the kitchen door.

Watch Out for Signs

Start spreading newspapers around the room just in case the puppy needs to go to the toilet really bad. Head bent down, sniffing is usually the most common sign that the pup is looking for a place to pee/poop. When you see this, invite the pooch over to the newspapers and encourage him to do his business there. If he manages to pee/poop exactly on the newspaper, praise him for a job well done and offer a treat. Do this continuously and pretty soon, the pooch will understand that going to the bathroom on the newspaper makes his owner happy.

Timing Is Everything

Of course, you can't expect the pup to use the newspapers as his bathroom forever! The newspapers are simply there as a "back up plan" just in case the pup finds himself really needing to go but no human to let him out. As the owner however, it's best to let the pooch out every day so that he can 'go' outside. The best time for this is in the morning before breakfast or at night after dinner. By maintaining a constant schedule of exercise-food-sleep, your pooch will enjoy regular bowel movements. This way, even if you leave him alone at home, you're 100% sure that there are no nasty surprises waiting.

Introducing the Crate

The crate is also another great tool to teach dogs' bowel control. Dogs naturally don't poop/pee where they sleep, hence their reluctance to use the crate as their bathroom. You can use this to your advantage by simply keeping the pup in the crate until it's time for them to go out. For example, if your schedule permits you to take the dog out for a bathroom break at 6 in the morning, make sure he stays inside the crate until 6AM rolls in. By doing so, he'd be able to wait until the proper time comes. Note though that the size of the crate matters. It should be just big enough for the pooch to circle in; otherwise if it's too big, it will still encourage pooping in the crate.

Pooping on Command

Some trainers like to teach their dog how to poop on command – something you can do as well. The trick is to wait for the pup to start circling, waiting for an area where he can do his business. Once you see him assuming the position, say your command word like "Doggy has to go!" making sure that the words are clear and distinct. Choosing unique words (something that probably wouldn't be said during a normal cause of events) would be best to ensure that the pooch doesn't get confused when out in public. Once the pup is done pooping, praise him for the achievement and provide a treat! Do this every time he poops where he's supposed to until the words and actions register.

Remember, part of being a responsible pet owner is picking up after your pup's poops! When out in public, make sure you're carrying a scooper or some tissue paper.

Chapter 5: What Breed of Dog Will Be the Best Fit for You?

Choosing the right breed of dog is like shopping at a supermarket. You have dozens of options to choose from. There are various factors you need to consider to ensure that you pick the proper breed of dog. The breed you choose largely depends on who is going to spend the most time with the dog. You also take into account the people who will be in constant contact with the dog. Are there babies or children in your home? This means that you have to look for a breed that's particularly friendly and safe to babies and small children.

Another important question you need to answer is what's your purpose in getting the dog? Are you going to train it to become a guard dog? This means you need to get one of the breeds that are known for their aggressiveness and guarding skills. Or maybe you just want a dog who will serve as companion for a senior citizen in your family. So, the question you need to answer is what are the best dog breeds for seniors? These are just some of the questions we are going to tackle in this chapter. I am going to help you look for the breed of dog that fits your lifestyle and addresses your personal preferences.

There are literally hundreds of dog breeds in the world today. The latest updated list from the World Canine Organization (WCO) shows that there are at least 340 recognized breeds of dogs. These breeds are divided into ten (10) groups based on the dog's appearance, size, function, and purpose.

These groups are as follows:

1. Sight hounds

2. Companion and toy dogs

3. Retrievers, water dogs, flushing dogs

4. Setters and pointers

5. Scent Hounds and related breeds

6. Spitz and primitive types

7. Dachshunds

8. Terriers

9. Pinscher and Schnauzer, Molossoid breeds, Swiss Mountain and Cattle Dogs and other breeds. Molossian breeds also include the dogs known as mastiffs by most other kennel clubs.

10. Sheepdogs and cattle dogs other than Swiss Cattle Dogs. This group includes the dogs classified as herding dogs by kennel clubs.

Factors to Consider

Here are the most important factors to take into account when looking for the appropriate dog breed for you:

1. The Size of the Dog

This is probably the most common consideration among folks who are planning to get a dog. Are you planning to get a small dog or a big dog?

Needless to say, bigger breeds require more space both inside and outside of your house for their exercise. Smaller breeds are more appropriate for smaller environments such as mobile homes, apartments, or senior care centers. They are perfect for those who simply want a little lap dog that they can carry around wherever they go.

However, you should be reminded that having a small size does not necessarily mean less care. There are some breeds that are small but are much more difficult to take care of compared to larger breeds.

Anyway, below is a quick overview of dog sizes and the breed examples that correspond to them.

- 1 to 10 pounds, X-Small: yorkies, Chihuahuas, Pomeranians, papilloma, Maltese dog breeds
- 11 to 25 pounds, Small: Brussels griffons, Chinese crested, Pekingese, Havanese, lhasa apsos, French bulldog, West Highland terriers, bichon frises, miniature pinschers, Boston terrier, poodles, dachshunds, cairn terriers, pugs, shih Tzu
- 26 to 40 pounds, medium: beagle, miniature schnauzer, Shetland sheepdogs, Scottish terriers, cavalier King Charles, American Staffordshire terriers
- 41 to 70 pounds, large: bull terriers, wheaten terriers, sharpies, Australian shepherds, spaniels, English springer spaniels, basset hounds, Welsh corgis, cocker spaniels, bulldogs, boxers
- 71 to 90 pounds, x-large: chow chows, border collie, standard poodle, Rhodesian ridgebacks, Airedale terriers, vizslas, collies, weimaraners, Siberian

huskies, Doberman pinschers, Rottweiler's, German shepherds, golden retrievers, Labrador retrievers
- 91 to 110 pounds, xx-large: Alaskan malamute, Bernese mountain dog, great Danes, weimaraners, St. Bernard's, Old English sheepdogs, malamutes

A good way to narrow down your list of breeds is to identify the size of dog that you want. To do this, you should take into account not just your preferences of size but also your current living situation. If you are staying in a tiny apartment, it will be problematic for a huge dog that can barely maneuver around the place. On the other hand, if you have a 10-acre yard, it will be hard to keep track of a small breed of dog that can easily get lost when it goes outside unattended.

2. Grooming and Climate Tolerance

Grooming is one of the most time-consuming tasks in taking care of a dog. Naturally, dog breeds with longer and thicker hair and coats are often more difficult to wash and groom. They also need to be washed more regularly. The more hair an animal has, the more grooming it requires per week.

Another important aspect that is in need of your consideration is the climate in where you live. Fluffy and long haired dog breeds usually have really low heat tolerance. With that said, it's probably not a good idea to get dogs with fluffy and long haired coats if you live in an area that has a really hot climate and daily weather.

On the same note, dogs with very short hair and coats have extreme low tolerance to the cold. If you reside in an area that is known for its cold weather, it's a good idea to ensure that the dog breed you pick can easily handle those freezing temperatures and snow. The good news is that there are a good number of cold climate dog breeds for you to choose from. These include the following breeds: Akita, Alaskan malamute, American Eskimo dog, Bernese mountain dog, Great Pyrenees, Keeshond, Saint Bernard, Samoyed, Siberian husky, and the Tibetan mastiff.

3. Activity Level of the Dog

Some dogs have more energy than others. You can usually determine a dog's activity level by its breed. For instance, the Pembroke Welsh corgi or the Shetland sheepdog is known for their insane activity levels. So, don't get a Shetland sheepdog if you think you won't be able to keep up with its level of activity. Energetic and active dogs are in need of routine exercise. If you know you cannot commit to an exercise routine for your dog, then you should probably not get a high-energy dog. You would be better off with a lower energy dog.

4. Coat Shedding

It's important to consider a dog's coat shedding because you or some members of your household may be allergic to dog hair and certain varieties of fur. Most of the allergies are caused by long haired dogs.

Excessive coat shedding can also turn into a matter of cleanliness and housekeeping. If you keep long haired dogs that shed substantial amounts of hair every single day, you may need to clean and vacuum the house every day.

As a general rule of thumb, dog breeds with longer and thicker coats shed a lot more compared to dog breeds with shorter coats.

Dogs with silky coats also shed less hair compared to dogs with wiry or curly hair.

5. Temperament

There are some dog breeds that are considered more friendly and outgoing while there are those that are more prone to display aggression. An aggressive dog may be what you are looking for if you want a guard dog or a very protective animal. On the other hand, if all you want is a family pet, then you should go for breeds that are more of the easy-going type.

Some of the most important temperament characteristics you should look into include compatibility with other animals, sensitivity, loyalty, intelligence, playfulness, activity level, energy, protectiveness, and aggression.

For example, gundog breeds such as Weimaraners were bred as working dogs and to be sociable. So, while they are quite intelligent, loyal and good natured, they tend to be anxious when left alone. If you live alone in a small apartment in the city and are away for several hours for work, you should look for another breed. Golden retrievers on the other end make excellent family pets because they are loyal, smart, and gentle.

6. Cost

Some dogs are more expensive to maintain compared to other dogs. The most common expenses associated with the upkeep of a dog include food and treats, water bowls, beds or bedding, collars and leashes, toys for outside and inside, crates for traveling, grooming supplies and kits, periodic vaccinations, veterinary care, and other health-related expenses.

You should also consider expenses for spaying, neutering, deworming, training, vitamins, supplements, training aid, and waste disposal. It's not uncommon to spend a few hundred dollars for a dog every single month.

7. Training Requirements

It doesn't matter what kind of puppy you get, you still have to do some training for it. But here's something you should know. Some dogs are more difficult to train compared to the others. However, this won't make any difference if you are bent on training your dog yourself.

If you think you won't have enough time for training once you get the dog, you should probably get a breed that doesn't require vigorous and routine training. Low-maintenance dog breeds include Dachshund, Greyhound, French bulldog, Chihuahua, cavalier King Charles spaniel, West Highland white terrier, and Brussels griffon.

8. Space Requirements

Some dog breeds require huge spaces where they can roam and get their exercise. Other breeds can survive even in limited and confined spaces. The point here is that you should get a dog that's suitable for the available space you have at home or at your apartment.

Another important thing to remember is that just because a dog breed is small does not necessarily mean that it needs little space. There are small dog breeds that are so active and energetic that they still require large spaces to be happy and healthy. On the same note, just because an it's a large breed does not always mean it needs a lot of space to roam. This is why it's important that you look into a breed's space requirements not on the size of the breed itself.

9. Exercise Requirements

How much exercise does my puppy needs? This is one of the most common questions that dog owners ask. First of all, different breeds have significantly different activity needs. Needless to say, active and very energetic dogs need to be taken out more often for exercise because they get depressed if they are inactive for too long.

The bottom line here is that all dogs need exercise for both their physical and mental health. You should take the time to learn and understand the exercise requirements of the breed you plan on taking home.

Picking a puppy to bring home should not be a rushed decision. Deciding to bring in a puppy into a home is like welcoming a new member of the family. You have to make sure that you have everything in place and ready before the puppy walks in through the door. Being prepared is the key to making sure that the puppy has a good start in life under your care.

In the following sections, I am going to make it even easier for you to find the right breed with our list of recommendations based on certain situations or based on what you need the dog for. For example, if you have kids in the house and you are looking for a breed that's friendly to children, we have the exact recommendation list for you. I don't claim these recommendation lists to be complete, but these lists should make an excellent start-off point. Anyway, you can find the right dog for your current situation if you just take the time to review your options. Use some of these lists to help you come up with your final decision.

Chapter 6: Physical and Mental Exercises for Your Dog

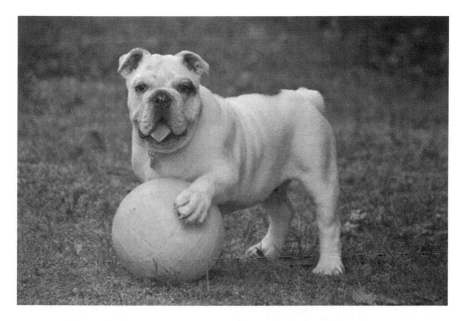

Dogs are just like their human masters. In order to function properly as they should, they need to be both physically and mentally healthy. They are like children. If you don't give them something to do, they will go and make their own fun. Dogs are meant to live very active lives. If they are not active enough, they get bored and all sorts of behavior problems can arise.

However, you also need to make sure that you're not subjecting your dog to excessive exercise. Dogs need exercise but too much exercise can harm them. Truth is told, according to the ASPCA, boredom and excess energy are two of the most common reasons behavior problems arise in dogs. This makes complete sense because dogs are supposed to live active lives.

It's simple, really. If you want a happy, healthy, and well-behaved puppy, you have to invest in activities that aim to improve the puppy's physical and mental well-being. Countless studies have shown over and over again that well-exercised dogs chew less, bark less, sleep more, behave better, and are easier to control.

So, what you need to do is to come up with your own physical and mental enrichment plan for your dog. You get a far happier pet if you stimulate their brain daily. Otherwise, they will get easily frustrated, bored, and they can even develop behavioral problems.

Below are some physical and mental exercises that you can use on your new puppy.

1. Give your dog some obedience training.

Obedience training is the type of exercise that's perfect for dogs because it stimulates both of the dog's physical and mental capabilities. Now, there are various kinds of obedience training. The ones you should use depend on the breed and size of the puppy you are training.

For example, obedience training for a Great Dane may be different from obedience training for a Chihuahua. Obedience training is a great way to develop a well-behaved dog. It also helps in building bonds between you and your dog.

2. Teach your dog new tricks.

Teaching new tricks to a puppy is one of the activities you should be regularly doing with your dog. It's a fun and entertaining way to engage the puppy and stretch his learning chops. Try to set aside time every day for a trick-learning session. There's a ton of new tricks that you can teach your puppy aside from the common sit, stand, and come. Just a quick search on Google will provide you with hundreds of new ideas for tricks.

3. Teach your dog to help with the chores.

Just like people, doing jobs can stimulate the physical and mental health of dogs. Be creative and train your dog to perform simple chores around the house like opening the fridge, taking the garbage bag outside, carrying groceries, closing the door, sorting the laundry, picking up the trash, or waking up the kids. Teaching your puppy to help with chores will give the dog something to do on a regular basis. The chores keep them occupied and exercised.

4. Teach your dog the names of their toys.

Teaching your puppy to identify the names of the toys it plays with is a fun activity and it keeps the dog thinking and mentally stimulated.

Begin with a favorite toy that your dog can easily recognize such as a ball. Give the ball a name. Just like any training technique, repetition is key here. Hold the toy, wriggle it, call the attention of your dog and say the name of the toy.

When the dog acknowledges the gesture, say yes. Keep on repeating this process until you get the reaction you want from the dog. Sooner or later, the dog will start identifying the toy with the name you provided for it.

5. Teach your dog how to put their toys away.

It's best to teach the dog how to do this after training it to identify with the names of the toys. Basically, you are going to train the puppy so that it puts away the toys back into the toy box after play time. This is why it's important that they should be able to identify the toys by name.

When you mention the name of a particular toy, the dog should pick it up and bring it back to the toy box.

Before you start with this exercise, you must be aware with the "take it" and "drop it" cues in dog training. You should have trained the dog first in responding to "take it" and "drop it" commands.

6. Train your dog on how to properly respond to clickers.

Clicker training is a very popular animal training method because it's effective and generates mostly positive results. Clicker training is especially great for training dogs because it's an effective method of positive reinforcement.

Clicker training starts by teaching the dog to associate the clicker sound with a treat. Whenever the clicker sounds, a treat is offered immediately for the dog. When the dog does the right thing, the clicker sounds, and a treat comes right after.

Keep on pushing this positive reinforcement until your dog gets the routine. When using a clicker for training, there are common mistakes you should avoid like clicking without treating, clicking too often, and sending mixed messages.

7. Teach your dog how to properly count.

It's time to push your dog's intellectual boundaries by teaching it how to count. It's definitely going to be difficult but it's possible. Science has shown that dogs have the ability to count if they are taught well. There are several methods on how to teach a dog to count. There's the "tell me method", the "eyes and hands method", and the "target counting method". Seek out the differences between these methods so that you can identify which method will suit the breed of dog you are going to train.

8. Create a scavenger hunt in the backyard or outside your house.

This is yet another game that both exercises the dog's body as well as stimulates their thinking prowess. Scavenger hunts can be fun, and you and your kids can even participate in it.

However, before you plan a scavenger hunt, make sure that you have taught the dog the concept of "find it". Teach the dog how to go looking for items like toys, treats, and food. The dog has to positively respond when you command it to go and "find it".

For example, you throw a chew bone into some brush then command your dog to go find it. If the dog has been properly trained with the "find it" command, it would go looking after the chew bone and bring it back to you. The same concept can be applied to treats and food.

9. Create an interesting food puzzle game for your dog.

There's a ton of food puzzle games being sold in the market that were specifically designed and developed for dogs. These puzzle games are very effective in physically and mentally exercising your new dog. These games require time, patience, and problem-solving skills from your pet. You can combine these puzzles and games to make them more challenging and interesting for your puppy. You can purchase these puzzles and toys from pet shops. If you don't find what you are looking for in your local pet store, you can always do your shopping online.

Food puzzle toys are usually made of hard plastic or rubber. They are in the form of containers with treats and food inside. Each end of the toy has holes where the food and treats are supposed to be dispensed. A dog must work by nibbling, licking, pawing, chewing, and shaking the toy to get the food out.

Some toys are more complicated than others. You should start with simpler food toys then slowly introduce more complicated toys and puzzles. Before buying a food puzzle toy, make sure that it's made from safe and non-toxic materials.

10. Come up with an indoor agility or obstacle course for your dog.

It takes time and a little bit of planning to set up an agility or obstacle course for your dog but it's worth it. Agility training is a great exercise for your dog. Going through a course that includes passing through a variety of obstacles will stimulate and challenge your dog's body and mind. The course strengthens its muscles, maintains its fitness, improves its coordination skills, and improves its endurance. The dog's natural instincts will also get a major boost. And of course, going through the agility courses will further strengthen the bond you have with your dog.

Most of the tools and materials you need to set up agility or obstacle course can be purchased at a pet shop or at a local hardware store. These include teeter boards, tire jumps, tunnels, pause tables, standard jumps; dog walks, and weaves poles.

You can set up the course in any way you want. If you are not sure how to get started, there are a lot of agility course maps that you can find online. Just download the maps and follow how the course has been set up.

11. Play hides and seek with your dog on a regular basis.

Teaching your dog to play hide and seek is an enjoyable workout for the dog's brain and body. It exercises the body because the dog is encouraged to move around and be active. It exercises the mind because the dog is forced to think and be creative in finding its master. You can play hide and seek anywhere where there's enough space for the dog to roam around. You can play it inside your apartment or in the backyard if you have one.

12. Play tug of war with your dog.

Dogs have that natural instinct to clamp their teeth and pull on things. In playing tug of war with your dog, it allows your pet to have an outlet for such urges. This is an activity that requires a lot of energy, so it works out the dog from head to toe.

There are various types of tug toys available in the market. They come in all sizes and shapes. The rope you get depends on the size and breed of your dog. Needless to say, small dogs require thinner ropes. You also need to train the puppy on how to properly play tug of war. Teach the puppy to respond to commands like "give" and "drop it".

13. Play fetch with your dog.

There are a lot of reasons to regularly play a game of fetch with your puppy. First, it encourages your dog to exert a lot of energy. And dogs enjoy playing the game.

Choose the appropriate toy because some dogs can be very particular about the toys they will play fetch with. Some dogs prefer balls while others prefer wooden sticks. Others prefer a Frisbee.

What you should do is experiment with several fetch toys and sees which toys excite your dog the most. Safety is a serious issue in this game so you should get a toy that isn't too small or too big for the dog.

14. Let your puppy sniff and explore during your daily walks.

Going for a walk is one of the most anticipated parts of a dog's life. You can use these daily walks to provide mental stimulation for your pet by letting it sniff around and explore its surroundings. You may look at walking as an exercise for your dog but your dog treats the activity as an exploration. That said, you should let him explore and have fun.

15. Play the shell game.

This is a fun and interactive activity that you and your dog can enjoy. The game involves hiding a treat under one of three containers, shuffling them, and letting the dog choose which container holds the treat. It's a powerful way to stimulate your puppy's brain and help it improve its problem-solving skills.

Again, this is a game that can only be played if you trained your dog how to play it. It's best to make use with a heavier container (i.e. clay) because it won't be that easy for the dog to trip it over. Drill a hole in each container to allow the puppy to be able to smell the scent of the treats inside.

A puppy needs mental stimulation and regular exercise to stay healthy physically and mentally. The physical exercises keep the dog fit and can possibly prolong the dog's life. The mental exercises keep the dog occupied and mentally alert. Mental exercises are also a great source of entertainment for the dog. Just like humans, dogs need fun and entertainment in their lives.

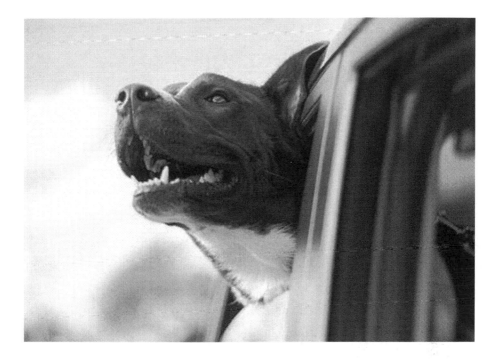

Chapter 7: Understanding Dog Psychology and How Their Minds Work

Before you start training your new puppy, it's important to have a clear understanding of how their psychology works and how they evolved from the wild wolves of yesterday to the modern dogs of today.

With that said, in this chapter, I will be providing you with a quick history lesson on the psychology and evolution of modern dogs. By dog psychology, I mean the overall behavior of dogs and why they behave in that or this way.

This is very important because properly training a dog begins with understanding the basic psychology of the pet. Needless to say, if you are aware of the basics of dog psychology, you can engage in better communication with your dog. Better communication translates to more effective training.

But First, How Did Modern Dogs Come About?

Truth be told, scientists are still putting the pieces together to get a clearer picture of how dogs came about and how they evolved to the breeds we have today. However, we already have an idea of how the process went about. Molecular evidence shows that dogs descended from a breed of gray wolf that was domesticated by prehistoric humans about 130000 years ago. This basically means that all dogs today have a common ancestor.

This may prompt you to ask why Poodles are so different from the Great Danes if they share a common ancestor. The scientific answer to this is that all modern dogs went through years and years of selective breeding. Experts often describe this as artificial evolution.

So, which of the dog breeds we have today are the oldest? Well, the general consensus for now is that the oldest breeds are the following: Afghan hound, Akita, Alaskan malamute, Basenji, Chinese Shar-Pei, Chow Chow, Saluki, Samoyed, and the Siberian husky. Scientists dated these dog breeds through meticulous research. They compared DNA from dozens of dogs and wolves, including ancient fossils. The pieces are slowly coming together but scientists still have a lot of work ahead of them before the exact evolution of dogs can be clearly understood.

But we know for sure that modern and domesticated dogs evolved from wild wolves that early humans caught and befriended. The moment the animal became friends with humans that are where the breeding began. And here we are today with nearly four hundred (400) breeds of modern dogs. This number will likely grow in the years to come as we continue to breed the animals.

The Psychology of Today's Modern Dog Breeds

The most important takeaway from our short history lesson about the evolution of modern dogs is that they have come from wild ancestors. This means that today's dogs still carry a lot of the characteristics and attributes of their ancient ancestors.

For example, these ancient dog ancestors were social pack animals. To this day, most dogs are by their nature still social pack animals. This explains why majority of dog breeds today tend to get along very well with other dogs even if the other dogs are from completely different breeds. No matter their breed, the social instincts of their ancestors still run in their blood.

This ancestry also explains why most dogs get along well with humans. We are social creatures just like them and their instincts often tell them to join our pack. For most dogs, they now see us as the leader of the pack. This is why they obey us, behaves well when they are around us, and is willing to do just about anything to please us.

In a dog pack, there are three key positions - the front, middle, and rear. The dogs in the front are the pack leaders and their responsibilities include finding what the pack needs to survive like food, water and shelter.

The dogs in the middle position are the mediators. They are not that strong or intelligent to become leaders but they are not that weak or sensitive to be relegated at the rear. The middle dogs help maintains peace and stability in the pack by policing themselves and the dogs at the rear. When you see two dogs fighting and a dog or two tries to break up the fight, the ones breaking up the fight are usually middle position dogs. They play a very important role in keeping the pack together.

The dogs in the rear are the most sensitive ones in the pack and their job is to alert the pack especially the leaders if they sense that the pack is in serious danger.

Not every dog in the pack can be a leader. It just doesn't work that day. There's the leader and then there's the followers. That's the dog hierarchy since the beginning of their evolution and that's not going to change anytime soon. It's important that you understand this dog pack hierarchy because as the owner and master of a dog, you are looked upon as part of the pack. Every dog needs leadership and since you are considered as the leader of the pack, you need to act like one. If a dog doesn't have strong leadership, it can become unbalanced. This might lead to anxiety, confusion, and aggression towards humans and other dogs.

Understanding Dog Pack Hierarchy and Why It Matters

Dogs are social animals with a well-defined pack hierarchy. Every dog that belongs to a pack has his own unique place in the social order. This is how wolf packs operate and always bear in mind that all modern dogs evolved from wild wolves. If this social order gets broken, members in the pack become confused and unstable. This is where most forms of conflict occur.

It's important that you are knowledgeable about this pack structure so that you can easily maintain your position as leader and master. If a dog starts losing faith in your leadership, it becomes aggressive and its behavior becomes problematic.

As the master of the pack, it is your job to set both the rules and the limitations for your dog. You are looked upon as the alpha leader. Your dog needs you to provide it with guidance on how it should behave. If your dog understands what you expect from it, a stable and happy relationship is established. This applies to all breeds of dogs.

All dogs are born with an instinctive sense of pack mentality. In a lot of cases, you can determine if a dog is going to be a leader or a follower as early as when it's still a puppy. If you have ever seen a litter of puppies and observed them as they grow up, you can see that some of them are more aggressive than the others. Some of the puppies tend to be able to control the behavior of the other puppies. As the puppies play and interact with each other, you can observe the ones with dominant personalities and the ones with submissive personalities. That's the pack mentality in action.

Building Boundaries

As the leader of the pack, it's also necessary that you give your puppy a set of rules, limitations, and boundaries. This is among the hallmarks of training a dog and making it behave appropriately. Your puppy has to know what it's allowed to do, where it can do it, and how long it's supposed to do it. It's also about teaching the puppy where it can go and where it can't.

Establishing boundaries is a good solution to various canine behavior problems like bolting out the door, begging at the dinner table, chewing on household items, and jumping on the furniture. In creating boundaries, you establish a line which your puppy will understand as a line that it's not supposed to cross.

1. Claim your space.

You have to do what real dog pack leaders do. Dogs establish their dominance through body language and actions. You need to do the same. If you don't want your puppy entering a particular room, you should stand on the door and block its way. If you don't want it jumping on the couch, stand over it.

2. Take the lead.

Never stop emphasizing that you are the leader of the pack. You should always be the first one to enter a room unless you command your dog to go ahead. You drive down the point that you are the leader and your dog is a follower.

3. Teach your dog how to wait.

Training your dog to be aware of its boundaries includes teaching it how to time its actions. This means providing the dog with signals when it's okay to do something or otherwise.

4. Correct the dog's behavior at the right time.

The best time to correct a dog and send the signal that it's about to commit improper behavior is when the dog is on the act of doing it. For example, you confront the dog just as it jumps on the couch not when it has already jumped on the couch. Correcting the puppy's behavior when it's already on the couch can create confusion in the dog.

5. Be consistent with your boundaries to avoid confusing your dog.

It takes time for a puppy to learn about its boundaries. You have to be consistent in the restrictions you impose upon your puppy.

In a nutshell, your puppy looks up to you for direction and protection. Showing it the boundaries for its actions lets it know what it can't do and where it can't go. Establishing boundaries is crucial during the dog's early years. Teach them as early as possible. It's harder to train dogs to respect boundaries if they are already adults.

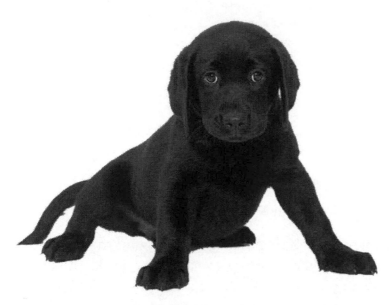

Establishing Routines

Most puppies will need a few weeks at the very least to learn house training routines. So don't be alarmed when other dog owners brag about needing just a few days for their pups to learn how to do their business properly.

To do this, you need to set a routine, and you have to be **very** consistent.

Here are some tips to help you out:

- **The Power of Delayed Gratification.** If you know anything at all about puppies, then you know that these dogs love to be cuddled and showered with affection. It seems like this their primary purpose in life. And you can use this **need for affection** to your advantage.

For example, when you release your pup from isolation or after he has taken his nap, one of the first things he will want to do is to find you and "reconnect" with you.

But you shouldn't give him what he wants right away. Instead, say your phrase for the bathroom area and direct him to it. Once your puppy has done his business correctly, you can then reward him with a cuddle. You can be affectionate, and you can talk to him, walk him, cuddle him in your arms, or even just greet him.

Your puppy will then realize that these things will happen **only** when he does his business in the bathroom area.

- **The Same Route.** It's not enough that you use the same area again and again for your puppy's bathroom. The same **routes** must also be taken. So, if he comes from a specific area of your home, the same routes must be used. Go through the same door every time, and other people in your home should also learn these routes. If the routes aren't clear, then draw a map and indicate the paths from each location to your pet's designated toilet.

The point of this exercise is to teach your puppy how to get to that area himself. So, it may be a good idea to use a leash and direct your puppy to that place on his own. Don't carry him each time, because then he will expect to be carried when he wants to do his business.

- **Staying in the Designated Bathroom.** A puppy may be tempted to sniff or wander around the area.

53

Don't let them. Then they may also try to get some affection from you. You have to harden your heart and ignore him **until** he does his business.

- **Word Cues.** Always use the same words ("PEE") when he is in the process of eliminating. Say it over and over. In a few weeks or months, your puppy can then figure out what to do when you utter the words.

- **Lavish Affection.** Once your puppy has done his business, it's time to give him the affection he so craves from you. Don't be cheap with the praise. Instead, shower him with affection with lots of greetings, praise, and cuddles.

Keep these guidelines in mind when you set up your routine.

Setting the Schedule

Now it's time for you to set up a schedule for your pup's potty breaks. Smaller and younger puppies have smaller bladders, so of course they will need to go on a break more often. Older puppies may hold out for longer.

Still, each dog is different, so the rules here aren't really hard and fast rules. They're more like guidelines to help you out.

Here are the ages of the puppies and the suggested number of breaks:

- 6 to 14 weeks old. **9 potty breaks**
- 14 to 20 weeks. **7 potty breaks**
- 20 to 30 weeks. **5 potty breaks**
- More than 30 weeks old. **3 or 4 potty breaks**

The number of potty breaks is **not** exact. For young pups, for example it may be as few as 8 potty breaks to as many as 10. But this guide can help you when you're trying to draw a schedule.

Here's an example of a schedule if you work at home and your designated bathroom area is outside the house:

1. **Wake up early in the morning**. Time to go out with your puppy.

2. **Puppy has breakfast**. Go to the bathroom after eating. In some cases when a puppy is not interested in the food for reason, take him out for a quick potty break before feeding.

3. Midmorning (10 AM or so). **Another potty break.**

4. **Lunch feeding**. Go after puppy is done eating.

5. Midafternoon (2 PM or so). **Another break.**

6. **Dinner (5 PM or so)**. Another trip outside after the meal is complete.

7. **Midevening**. It's time for another trip. Meanwhile, don't offer him water after this time.

8. **Right before you go to bed**. Time for a curtain call, so to speak.

9. **In the middle of the night**. You may have to take him out again when he needs to do his business.

Now if you work outside your home, do not even think that your puppy can hold it in until you get home. There's no way this can happen, so if you can't be home then another person may have taken your place. It may be possible to use a special area for him that he can use when you're not at home, but that can be confusing for the puppy if you expect him to go out on his own to do his business.

A small room is fine too.

The idea is to have an easily accessible bathroom space for him to go to on his own, which you can then clean up easily too. You can lock away that particular bathroom space when you're home, so that the outside designated area will be used instead.

As you can see, owning a puppy requires 100% commitment from you. It's not surprising that many owners try to time the arrival of a new puppy with some sort of extended vacation. The bond you forge in the first few days and weeks can be strengthened if you spend more time with your pup.

Transitioning to Solo Bathroom Breaks

After a week or so of daily trips together to his special bathroom area, you can start making a transition. Encourage him when he makes his signals or uses a bell to communicate his needs. Repeat the word "outside" (or whatever word you've chosen for the bathroom area) and praise him. Then put him on a leash and lead him to the bathroom area.

Repeat all these steps for different rooms, starting with the nearest room to the designated area. Then you can range even farther and farther along to different areas in your home.

Once you leash him, you can now start to drop the leash 75% of the way to the bathroom area, and see if he can find it on his own. Once he does this with some consistency, you can begin dropping the leash halfway to the designated area. Then you can drop it at the 25% mark.

It's a bit like teaching a child to ride a bike, doesn't it? You have to be there in the beginning, and then you cut off the need for your presence gradually. You start by being there to praise him when he does his business, and afterwards he'll do it on his own and you can cuddle with him when he does it correctly and comes back to you.

Understanding Your Puppy's Signals

There's really no need for a Star Trek Universal translator to understand your puppy. Just keep in mind that a puppy is basically a baby. And like a baby, you will know when it's time for him to go do his business. Puppies have their own ways of telling you. Some dogs may be barkers, although pups are usually not. Others may start nipping you to get your attention.

Now there's no point in correcting this kind of behavior, really, just like it's pointless to correct six-month-old baby who's crying. Just make sure you recognize the behavior so you can be ready. Often it's all about sniffing for a place and then circling that area before he starts squatting. You'll need to be very attentive so you can reduce the number of "accidents."

You can also try teaching him how to ring a bell when he needs to go out. Every time you lead him to the area, pass a bell that's low enough for your puppy to reach. Ring the bell each time you go to the special bathroom. Then encourage him to ring the bell himself before you go to the bathroom. Every time he rings the bell, take him to the bathroom and reward him with cuddles and treats.

If your pup still doesn't understand, before he wakes up in the morning you can smear the bell with some butter or cheese. Once he licks it, you **immediately** go to the special bathroom. By doing this kind of training, he will be more inclined to ring the bell every time he needs to pee or poop.

Chapter 8: Choosing Your Pup's Bathroom Location

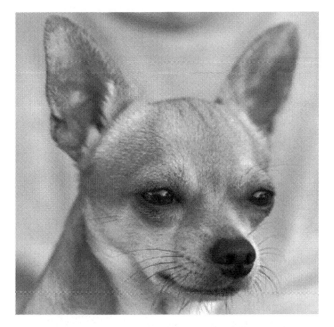

The jury's still out on whether you should have your pup's special bathroom inside or outside. In general, outside is always a good idea although for puppies that may not be practical. Puppies shouldn't be too hot or too cold, and your chosen area should be private as well as shaded from the sun.

Puppies are good for inside bathrooms because they aren't all that big. This is especially true if you live in an apartment.

The basic restrictions are the same for indoor bathrooms.

1. You use the same spot consistently, and you take the same routes.

2. Use the same word for the area, such as "toilet", "bathroom", or "papers". The word paper is popular because you usually use a piece of paper for that bathroom.

3. When your pup is doing his business, keep repeating the same words such as "do your business" for the activity.

4. When you bring him to the inside bathroom, you also withhold your affection until he does his business. You cuddle him **after** the deed is done.

5. The special bathroom should not be an area where you spend a lot of time interacting with your puppy. It should be for one purpose only.

6. It should be far enough from his feeding area, and also preferably far enough from his sleeping quarters. But it should be accessible.

7. It should have some measure of privacy, and the surface should be non-absorbent.

Having both Inside and Outside Bathrooms for Your Puppy

Is this possible? Can your puppy actually learn to use two different bathrooms?

It all depends on your dog, of course. But it may be possible for your puppy to learn this. After all, there may be times when going outside to do his business may not be convenient.

For example, the weather may not be conducive for outdoor activities of any kind. So what you can do is to teach your puppy to use the indoor bathroom when you have paper in hand, and to go outside when there's no paper.

Puppies are not exactly fast learners, so this can be a bit more difficult than you think. But it is possible. You just need to be clear about what you want. And that is for him to do his business "on paper" when you're not around or when the weather is bad, and to go outside at other times.

You just need to be consistent, which is somewhat ironic considering you're trying to teach a dog to go to two different bathrooms.

But here are some other suggestions:

- Take him to the outside toilet whenever you're home. You only use the indoor toilet when the weather is really bad.

- Teach him the bell trick, so that you know when your puppy wants to do his business. You then take him to either the outdoor or indoor bathroom with the paper.

- When no one's around, secure your puppy in a small playpen in which there's an area with papers for him to use. You can use **Bulldog ology Puppy pads**, and you can clean these pads in front of your puppy. This emphasizes the lesson of eliminating only in the designated bathroom.

- As much as possible, the location of the indoor bathroom should also be in the way of the outdoor bathroom. You can then keep on repeating the same word ("papers", for instance) when you lay the papers down.

- During his scheduled potty breaks, you can wait for 5 minutes for your puppy to do the deed. If it's not yet done in that time, you may leash or crate your dog for about 5 to 15 minutes before you try it again. You can also watch out for his business signals during the waiting time. This can also train your puppy to "hold it" a little longer by building his bladder muscles.

Remember, whether or not you use the indoor or outdoor facilities, you need to make sure you pick up after your dog. In some places, this is actually the law. You can buy some poop scoopers in pet stores, or you can just use a plastic bag as a glove, pick up the stuff, and then turn the plastic bag inside out. With plastic bags, you have no real excuse not to pick up after your dog when you go out.

Chapter 9: Correcting Behavior Problems

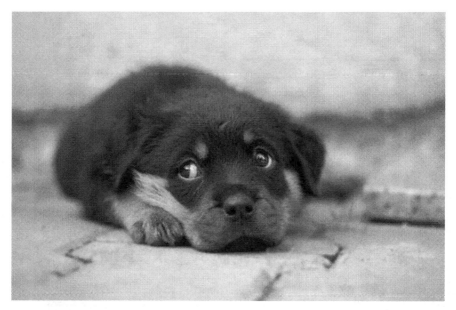

You have a puppy. Let's face it, there will be a lot of naughtiness around your house, and that is all normal. Puppies have a lot to learn on their way to becoming adult dogs, and that includes testing your limits and pushing the boundaries to see how far you will actually let them go.

Bad behavior is part of the deal of adopting a puppy. You should be aware that it is in your puppy's nature to show over excitement in ways you find unacceptable. Just like it is a natural thing to be stressed. It is your job to pin-point the reason for the bad behavior, eradicate the culprit, and completely redirect your puppy with nothing but love and understanding.

Correcting behavioral problems requires time and patience, but approaching the issue with an exaggerated reaction can set both you and your puppy to a path that is much harder to come back from.

Shushing the Barker

Having a constant barker in your home is no fun. Being robbed from your good night's sleep is nothing but a headache. But before you try to find a way to shush your barking ball of fur, you first need to determine what makes your pooch bark in the first place. Barking is a dog's way of communicating, and it is how they express themselves. See what your pooch is trying to tell you before you take a step further:

Barking for Attention

Your puppy just has to go through a phase of not being able to bear being alone. It is a normal part of their development. If your puppy is a loud barker when you are preparing to leave the house, here are some tips that may help you solve the problem:

-        Do not give them attention. By soothing a protester, you only add fuel to the fire. You will not only make things worse, but you will end up with a spoiled pup.

-        Do not leave or enter your house in a grandiose way because they are too exciting for your pup and they're only encouraging the barking even more.

-        Grab a hollow bone that is safe for your pup to chew on and fill it with some peanut butter. Offer it to your pup before you leave the house to keep them occupied.

    You can also try this:

1. Grab an empty can and put it in your pocket.

2. Get ready to leave the house and stand in the hallway.

3. Chances are, your puppy is already barking their lungs out. Throw the can toward (NOT AT your puppy). The goal here is for them to think that this reaction comes from the environment, not you.

4. When your puppy stops barking, give them attention.

5. Do this for every arrival and departure, until it realizes that stopping means getting the attention.

Barking at Everything

If your puppy is a real barker, then chances are, nothing in your home goes unnoticed. But, living with everlasting barking can be a real pain. If nothing is wrong with them, and you know that it is just an incessant barker, then know that the reason it is doing that is probably because it wants things to go away. For instance, if it barks at a cat, the cat will most likely go away. But if it starts barking at the postman, it may realize that their superpowers aren't as effective. So it will start barking some more and more. And then louder and louder.

If your first thought is to try yelling at them to stop (which is quite understandable given that his barking has become the soundtrack of your life), you will only make things worse. To dogs, yelling is the human way of barking. If you start yelling, they will only think that you are barking too, and that will lead to – that's right – more barking.

There are three things you can do to try to solve this issue:

1. Start (or intensify) training. Your pooch most likely thinks it is the leader and gets ego boosts as he is probably thinking that is his duty to guard the territory. By starting or devoting to a more intense training routine, you will let them know that it is actually you who is in charge of the home and that there are some rules to be followed.

2. Block off lookout posts. If your pup spends a lot of time in front of the window, guarding and keeping eye on things, make sure to block his access. If necessary, crate them more or secure them with a lead that is long enough for them just to lie down comfortably. Increase freedom gradually as your pooch becomes less interested in barking.

3. Avoid leaving them alone outdoors. If your pooch is confined and unsupervised for longer periods of time, that will only lead to territorial behavior and allow for boredom to swoop in, both of which are usually followed with long and loud periods of barking.

If neither of these seems to do the trick, maybe you can start teaching him new words. Teaching him Speak and Quit may help you put a stop to their excessive barking:

1. First, you need to teach your pup that Speak means start barking. To begin this, simulate a visitor. Knock on the door or ring the bell. Make sure that your pocket is filled with doggy treats.

2. The second your pup starts barking say **"Speak"** in a firm tone.

3. Praise and reward them immediately.

4. Does this for a couple of days, until your puppy learns what speak means?

5. Once your pup starts barking when you give them the speak command, it is time to teach them to be quiet. Instruct your pup to "**Speak**".

6. Once it starts barking, say **"Quiet"** in a firm tone.

7. Wait for your pup to stop barking. If needed, say **"Quiet"** again.

8. It may take a while for your pup to stop barking, and that's okay. The second it stops, praise them like crazy and give it a treat.

9. Respond for as long as it takes for your pooch to learn that quiet means stop barking.

Once your pup learns that, you can use this command to shush them whenever their barking starts getting just a bit too much.

Not Accepting Biting

In the first couple of weeks, biting is a normal daily hassle. But while soft mouthing is okay when your pup is playing with you, for some people, it can be a scary, if not a traumatic experience. It is extremely important for you to teach your puppy that their razor-sharp teeth are not made for the human skin while it is still a young pup in order for them to learn right from the start what it cannot play bite with. Not to mention that this may prevent future injuries and even save you from a big fat lawsuit.

This training technique will discourage your pup to bite your skin as a part of its games:

1. Place one of your hands in your pup's mouth and shake it gently until it realizes that you want to play with them.

2. Play with your pup for a while. As long as it is soft mouthing you and doesn't apply pressure, let them have his fun. The second you feel their teeth piercing a bit sharper, say **"Ouch"** or another negative word, take your hand out, and stop playing with them.

3. Step aside, look away, and do not interact with them for about 30 seconds. Do this for about 5-6 times a day.

4. If your pup doesn't let go of your hand the second you say "Ouch", leave the room immediately and do not let your pup see you for a couple of minutes.

5. When your pup finally realizes that ouch means that it is time to let go of the hand, you can start teaching them that they shouldn't play biting with humans under no circumstances.

6. It may take a while for you to get your pup to realize that it shouldn't play biting at all, but you should be patient. To start, simply play with your dog and keep your hand close to its mouth, however, do not place it inside.

7. Wait until your pup starts biting. The second it touches your skin with its teeth, even if it is super gently, say **"Bad Boy/Girl"** or another similar word, get up, and stop interacting with them for a couple of minutes.

8. Do this every time their teeth meet your skin. This way they will eventually learn that biting is unacceptable.

Getting Chewing Under Control

You cannot exactly train your pup not to chew on things, and you should not even try. Chewing is not only a natural instinct and an interesting way to spend their time, but it also contributes to their physical and mental health. By chewing, your pup supports the flow of antibacterial saliva and keeps his gums and teeth stay healthy and strong. That is why appropriate chew toys can jumpstart the healthy development of puppy's permanent teeth and make the whole process a lot less painful.

However, just because it is supposed to chew on things doesn't mean that your new sofa should be all chewed-up. Besides providing rubber toys, appropriate ropes, and marrow bones, there are also some other tricks that can help your pooch keep his teeth away from your possessions:

-       Allow plenty of exercise. Most dogs start a chewing contest when they are bored or when they have a fair amount of extra energy that they have to channel somewhere. If you don't want your couch to be that place, make sure to take your puppy on longer walks in order to knock down their urge to chew on things inside the house.

-       Use taste deterrents. Taste deterrents are nasty-tasting liquids sold in spray bottles that you can use to discourage the pup from chewing on things. You can find them in most pet stores, and they are pretty cost-effective as your pup will not like the idea of chewing on something that tastes awful. These deterrents usually have no scent at all, so you shouldn't worry about having an unpleasant smell spreading inside your house. Bitter apple is a great choice for a taste deterrent.

When you notice them chewing on something inappropriate, simply grab the spray bottle and spray that object immediately, and let them notice you. After doing so, offer them a safe toy that they can chew on to encourage appropriate behavior.

-        Play a "No" and "Good Boy/Girl" game. Lay out several objects on the floor, among which you will place a couple of chew toys. Wait for them to grab an object. If it is an appropriate chewable, say "Good Boy/Girl". If not, say "No" to let your puppy know it should let go of the object.

-        Praise them. In many cases, puppies are encouraged to chew on their toys when they are encouraged to do so. Whenever you see them chewing on their toys, praise them to mark the good behavior, and then give them a treat as a reward.

Stopping the Digging Frenzy

If those muddy paws freak you out, relax. You need to learn to accept this behavior as a part of the normal canine instinct. But just because it is natural, it doesn't mean that it is okay for your pup to be passing their time turning your backyard into a construction site. Whether your puppy is fussy, stressed, or just bored, you will need to find a way to make them learn that digging whenever and wherever he feels like it is not acceptable.

Although just like chewing, you cannot exactly train them not to dig. However, there are a few tricks you can do that will discourage this action. The very first thing is to offer a digging spot for your puppy:

1. Pick an area in your backyard that your puppy can use for digging. Make sure to mark the territory so it's easy to distinguish where it's ok to dig and where it's not. If you leave in an apartment, you can provide a sandbox for digging in your bathroom from time to time, or you can even do this with a certain spot in the nearest park.

2. Bring toys to that spot, or even better, bury treats there to encourage your pup to be digging there.

3. Take your pup to that spot on a daily basis and encourage them to dig by instructing her **"Go Dig"** or another command by your choice.

4. When you catch your puppy in the act of digging someplace else, correct with a firm **"No"**.

You can also give some other tricks a try:

-        Dogs really dislike the citrus scent. Putting lemon or orange peels in the holes will most likely discourage your pooch from digging there.

-        To help your pup learn that digging in certain areas in your yard is not acceptable, you can install some sensors such as sprinkles there.

-        Do not spray your pooch with a hose when you catch them in the act. This is a common correction method that many dog owners use, however, this is not only cruel, but it will also make him dig even more if it gets all fussy. Instead, you can try burying some of its own feces. Dogs usually hate the smell and taste of their own feces, so give this a try if nothing else helps.

- Many dogs dig excessively when they are left alone. If that is the case, see if you can leave your pup indoors when leaving the house for a couple of hours.

Discouraging the Jumper

Dogs are social animals. It is in their nature to seek and give attention, as well as to show excitement and lavish us with love when we enter the door. Isn't that one of the main reasons why most people adopt puppies in the first place? Having a small pup jumping up every time he lays eyes on you is cute, but if this behavior is left unchecked, this can easily turn into a 60-pound force trying to knock you over. And that is something that you will begin dreading.

Jumping up is one of those behaviors that dog owners love to hate. Why? Because they usually start as a cute thing that the pup gets rewards for, and then quickly turn into something that can cause an injury to both the dog and the owner. So, what am I trying to say here? Never encourage a pup that is jumping up by rewarding the behavior. And I am not only talking about a reward in the form of a tasty treat. When a pup is jumping up, the reward it is seeking for is your attention. Rob it from that and they will soon stop performing the action that does not elicit the favorable outcome.

Turning Away from the Jump

When your pup jumps, the best response is to simply turn away from it. It may be heartbreaking not to give your pup attention when it is so excited to see you, but this is the most effective way to teach him to control their emotions, and believe me, once it grows into an adult dog, this trick you're teaching them now will be greatly appreciated.

Bring your hands to your chest and avoid eye contact. Once your pup sees that it gets no response, it will soon settle down. Once it is four-on-the-floor, praise them for being calm and reward them with your attention now.

Use Commands

If your pup has already mastered the "Sit" command, you can use this to get it to settle down. Again, as soon as it is on the floor, praise and reward immediately.

Go Out the Door

When you enter your door and you see your pup all excited and jumping up, simply open the door, step aside, and then close the door. Wait for your pup to calm down before going back inside. If your pooch starts jumping up again, repeat this process. Now, this may take a while, but don't lose faith. Your pup will soon pick up that you will not go through unless it greets you in a calm way. Once it does that, praise them like crazy and reward them with your attention. Or a smelly treat. No dog has ever refused that.

Chapter 10: Methods of Housebreaking

There are two main ways to housebreak your new puppy: paper training and crate training. Crate training is one of the quickest ways to housebreak your pup but not the best method if you must leave your pup for a longer period of time than your pup is able to hold it. For people who must work all day or be away for long periods of time, I recommend a combination of both methods.

Paper Training

The paper-training method is where you use newspapers and encourage your puppy to use these for going to the bathroom. You can also use special 'wee wee' pads that are scented with a chemical that attracts the puppy to use them. You can get these at any local pet store. They can make training easier, but they can be more costly as well. If you intend to continue using the pads, make sure you start with them and not paper. Don't mix newspaper and pads or your results will be very inconsistent.

The first thing you want to do is choose a confinement area, either in a very small room or a room that you can enclose with baby gates. Most people choose a bathroom, laundry room or kitchen area because these rooms are usually covered in tile or other flooring that is easy to keep clean. The confinement area should only be big enough for your pup's bed, food and water bowls, and his designated potty area.

There should be no visible floor space in the confinement area. The floor should have the bed or crate in one section, and newspapers or pads should cover the rest of the space. By using a small area, you are encouraging your pup to use the covered area of the floor to relieve himself. This will get him used to doing his business on the newspapers or pads. He won't potty in his bed or where he eats for reasons we have already discussed, and since it's the only other space available, the potty area becomes a natural choice. The instincts that Mother Nature gave him will guide him away from his 'den' area to eliminate.

When he does soil on the newspapers, try to clean them up as quickly as possible. You may want to consider leaving a rag that has a little of his urine on it in the designated spot to help him recognize where he's supposed to go, if you're using newspaper. The pads are already scented to attract the puppy to go there. There are also house-training sprays you can buy at any big pet store that serve the same purpose. The pheromones in them attract puppy back to the right spot. These sprays can also be used outdoors if you want to direct him to a certain area.

Once your pup becomes accustomed to potting on the newspapers, you can make the covered area smaller. You should have noticed which section of the area he has used most often, and keep all that section well covered. Start uncovering the area very close to his crate/bed and bowls. The goal is to continuously limit the designated 'inside potty area' by making the papered area smaller and smaller at the same time giving him frequent access to his 'outdoor potty area'. Therefore, it's important that you spend as much time as possible with your puppy so you can get him to his outdoor area as often as possible.

The key to quick and successful housebreaking when using the paper training method really depends on how much supervised training you spend with your pup. The more times you can get him outside to do his business and reward him, the quicker he will learn.

Crate Training

The second method of housebreaking involves the use of a crate. You want to make sure the crate isn't too large—it should be just big enough to fit a sprawled sleeping puppy. As discussed earlier, dogs do not like to urinate or defecate in their sleeping areas or dens. Once pups are safely mobile, their mothers push them outside so they can go potty.

Crate training helps puppies learn how to control their bladder and bowels. Ideally you should take a puppy outside about every hour to start. Gradually lengthen the time between trips, within the limitations of his little bladder. It's important that you keep your eye on the clock. You don't want to lose track of the time and force your puppy to go in his crate. The more he can feel positive that you'll let him out to relieve him in a timely fashion, the more incentive he has to wait for you. He wants praise from his pack leader, but he also needs to feel that he can trust you and rely on you.

When your puppy is not crated, watch carefully for signs that he needs to go out. Most dogs have a 'pre-potty' ritual of sniffing, circling, whining, etc. that he'll use to try to let you know what he needs. With a little observation, and a few accidents, you'll learn your dog's potty signals. Once that starts, pick him up and get him outside or onto paper (or a piddle pad) right away. You also need to understand that he can stop his urine, but once he starts a poop, leave him be. He can't control it and, if you try to move him to a better spot, you'll have a trail to clean up instead of a pile.

There are certain times that all puppies need to go out, so learn these times and avoid accidents.

- Immediately after waking up, in the morning or from a nap

- After any excitement or play

- Within 10-30 minutes of eating

- After a big drink of water

- The absolute last thing before bed at night

Carry the puppy outside to prevent accidents between the crate, or wherever you are, and the doorway. Some pups anticipate a bit too much and they'll go right in front of the door, seconds away from being in the correct spot. So, provide 'taxi service' for a little one. Also, unless they're truly desperate (or scared), most puppies won't pee on you. After all, you're Mom and Alpha rolled into one!

Whenever the puppy is inside the home, but cannot be directly supervised, he should be placed in his crate. A good time would be when you're cooking, watching TV, taking a shower or even away from the house for a short period. Take your pup out right before crating him, and again as soon as you let him out of the crate.

Another way to keep your puppy supervised but still be able to do things is to use 'tethering'. Basically, you attach him to you via his leash, so he goes where you go. This gives you the freedom to get some housework done. Alternatively, you can tether him to something like a table leg if you're going to be staying in one room of your home, for example, cooking. You need to keep a close eye on him still, and be prepared to drop what you're doing if he shows signs of thinking about going potty. Tethering does, however, give him time outside the crate to stretch, investigate, and learn. It's a great option when you're on the patio or deck, or if you're in the yard. Never let the pup roam unsupervised in the yard, even if it's securely enclosed. They will try to eat anything! I had one little guy who devoured a squished frog, bones and all, before I could stop him, and another who insisted on trying to eat acorns. Needless to say, both experienced severe 'gastric distress.' You also should know that many decorative plants are toxic to dogs.

You definitely want to crate your puppy at bedtime. Sleeping alone is probably a new experience for him, and a slightly scary one. Puppies generally sleep in a pile, the whole litter snuggled close together with their mother. You can ease the transition for your pup by giving him a stuffed toy to curl up with as a fake littermate and, if he's very young, a well-wrapped hot water bottle under the bedding. The ticking of a clock placed nearby can help to mimic the sound of Mom's heartbeat and it reassures many pups. Also, putting a piece of clothing that you've worn into the crate with him can calm his fears since he can cuddle up to your smell. A little consideration for his sudden sense of isolation at night can make it much easier for both of you to get some sleep!

Expect your puppy to have to go potty in the middle of the night for a while, so put his crate in or very near your bedroom if at all possible. He's still a baby after all! It's a good idea if you are proactive about getting him out by setting an alarm clock. Keep whatever shoes, coat, keys, etc., that you'll need when taking him out laid out ready to grab and go for those middle of the night jaunts. Have his leash pre-attached to his collar, so you can just snap the collar on him, or use a slip lead. These trips will only be necessary until he's 5-6 months old. As he gets older, he'll sleep longer, have more control over his bladder, and begin to wake you if he really needs to go. Within a few months, he'll be sleeping through the night without a problem.

The ultimate goal of crate training is to never let your pup go potty in the house. This requires that you (or someone) be there to take him out on time, so you need to fit that into your schedule without fail. If you must be gone more than five hours, use the paper-training method while you are away and set up a managed confinement area with his crate in it.

When done right, there are many advantages to crate training. Crate training can effectively teach a puppy that when the urge to go pee or poop occurs, they are capable of holding it (within their limitations of course). It fits wonderfully with their natural instincts as well. Crate training also strengthens the alpha-pack bond that you are building with your puppy. He is learning that he can rely on you to see to his needs; therefore, he feels he can trust you and have respect for his pack leader. This is the main reason why puppy owners who use crate training have found it to be a quicker way of not only housebreaking their pup, but also teaching other desirable behaviors.

Litter Pan Training

As mentioned earlier, litter pan training is growing in popularity. Many dogs take to it very well, and it provides an easier cleaner indoor option than just a space on the kitchen floor. For dog owners living in high-rise buildings, people with limited mobility, or dogs who are unsuited for the weather where they live, pan training allows ease and comfort for both owners and dogs. A dog trained to a litter pan will still potty outdoors when going 'walkies,' but he has another option as well. Since little dogs need to go more often than their bigger cousins, it's very helpful for them to have an acceptable indoor area where they can relieve themselves while their owners are away from home. Eight hours for a large dog is like 'holding it' for 24 hours to a little guy! Not a very reasonable expectation.

If a litter pan of some type is your chosen route, make sure you have it ready to go before beginning house-training. Find a convenient spot in your home to place it, and don't move it around except when you need to set up a confinement area. Your puppy needs to learn where to find it! You can relocate it once he's trained.

If your dog is not a toy breed, you'll need to provide a larger pan as he grows. Many people start with a traditional dog litter pan and change to a round one, since dogs like to circle before pooping. For a larger dog, this could even be something like a 'kiddie pool', perhaps moved into the garage or basement after he's trained.

Make sure that your dog can easily enter the pan without climbing or jumping. It needs to be simple for him to get in and out! You may need to cut the entryway down a bit lower so that he can step in. Some people like the pellets that are sold as litter, and there are several different types, and others just use a piddle pad in the pan. If your pup doesn't seem to like it, or tries to eat it, change to a different type of absorbing medium. [Cat litter doesn't work very well for most dogs because it really gets stuck in their feet.] The fake grass models have a tray underneath which collects the urine, but many folks like to line that with wee wee pads for quicker, easier cleaning.

Be aware, if you're not already, that although young male pups squat, as he matures he'll lift his leg to urinate. By that time you need to make provisions so that he doesn't pee over the top of the pan or onto the wall. You can purchase posts or little plastic fire hydrants, scented with attractant, to give him something to aim at, or use a pan with higher sides. If you have multiple dogs, you may need multiple pans. They sometimes don't want to share and won't use a pan that's already been soiled.

To train your pup to a litter pan, **follow the same procedures as crate training**. You just take the pup to the litter pan instead of taking him outside to the yard. If you need to be away for a while, set up a confinement area with the litter pan inside, just as you would do with paper training. Be sure to cover the rest of the floor with paper (in case of accidents) until your pooch is reliable with the pan!

Just as with newspaper, pads, and even the yard, the litter pan should be kept as clean as possible. Clean up messes as soon as possible, and change the litter following the instructions that come with it. Empty the pan for a thorough cleansing with disinfectant cleaner at least once a week, and hose off the plastic turf as well.

Crazy Training Plan

If you would like to streamline the housebreaking process, and you can completely free yourself from any other responsibilities, work or family, for a couple of days, then this 'extreme' method might be just the thing for you. It's very effective and creates a strong bond, but it does take its toll on you. If, like me, you're a bit of a risk-taker, read on.

The 'crazy' way to house-train your pup, within his physical bladder limits of course, is to be **completely proactive**. The pup *never* goes on the floor, not once. How do you achieve this miracle, you ask? With self-sacrifice and a total focus on the task, allowing no distractions. It's just you, puppy, and housebreaking.

This will work with a litter pan or a pad as well as going outdoors. It's actually a simple procedure, a sort of 'extreme crate training,' but you have to 'suck it up' and follow through—that's the craziness. It's 24/7 on your part until you reach his physical limits. After that, you never ask him to exceed those limits.

Still with me? Then here's how it goes. You bring puppy home and let him potty before you bring him inside. Ten minutes later, you take him out again (or take him to the pan or pad). Praise a successful trip! If he doesn't go, give him another ten minutes and then out again. After each successful potty break, you add five minutes to the time between trips, so you'd wait 15 minutes and then go out again. After each unsuccessful trip, repeat the same interval.

You need to continue this all day and all night, following and adjusting the schedule. Wake up (use an alarm), wake him up (really), and go out. (I slept on the sofa by the door to facilitate the process, while puppy slept tethered on the floor next to me.) Work some playtime in between some of the trips, and don't forget to wedge in some food for both you and the pup. Watch some TV together. But keep track of the time! You'll become a little zombie-like, but that's OK. Think of it as a short-term extreme sporting event. Stay focused on your mission!

A three-month-old pup will settle into a 3-4 hour maximum interval between trips. Once you know what that limit is for your pup, you can make arrangements to let him relieve himself within that interval. You can also crate him and crawl into bed until your next puppy potty break (set the alarm!).

Although you'll need about a day to fully recover, depending on what time of day you brought him home and started the process, you'll also have a very accurate idea of his bathroom habits and needs. You will have learned his potty rituals—does he sniff or circle, or both? (This can help you prevent future 'accidents' if he needs to go earlier than usual for some reason.) You've earned his trust, and he can count on you to meet, even anticipate, his needs. He's never eliminated anywhere except where you, his pack leader, have approved, so he won't be inclined to start. Even young as he is, he'll come to you for a potty break. And, in spite of the sleep disruption, it is time spent working together that can give you a very strong bond with your dog. Packs work cooperatively for the good of all, and that's what you two have just done together!

The follow-up is simply assuring that you never expect him, or force him, to exceed his capabilities. You get him to his designated area within his time limit, period. If you can't be there to do it, then you find someone who can help you out. This means at night, too! Set the alarm, take him for his potty break, praise, and go back to bed. Once he's 6 months old or so and has full control of himself, he'll be **extremely** reliable (and sleeping through the night).

Chapter 11: Top Techniques to Train your Dog

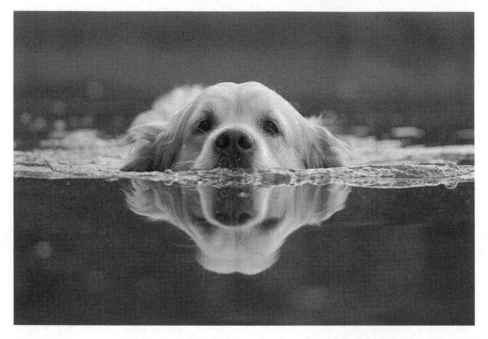

Make Use of his Paws

Teach your dog to shake your hand and give you a high five by following the steps listed below.

•   Let your dog sit across you.

•   Wait for him to lift his paws then use the clicker and give him a treat. Repeat this process for at least 4 to 5 times.

•   Whenever he lifts his paw, make sure to give a command by saying the word "Paw" then use the clicker and give him a treat so he could associate these actions together.

Jump

You can teach your dog how to ju

- Bring out your training stick

- Automatically, your dog w has to jump—and that is wh~

- If your dog doesn't jump, t~ the stick then when he touches it, angle ~ use the clicker and give him a treat.

- Then give a command by saying the word "jump" as you angle the stick higher once more. When he does jump, make sure to use the clicker and offer him a reward.

- Repeat until he no longer has a hard time jumping.

Teach him How to Leap

Leaping is another skill that will be very beneficial for your dog and that he can easily learn if he knows how to come to you. Here is what you have to do:

- Allow your dog to sit on the floor then carefully place a stick on the ground.

- Now, go to the other end of the stick and call the dog by his name.

- Use the clicker and give your dog a treat as he crosses the stick.

- Practice some more, then angle the stick even higher by placing it over stacks of books.

nd give him a treat upon doing so.

an

ons! Now you have reached the final week of
his time, you can teach your dog how to be reliable
like a person - or something like it. You see, a well-
ed dog is a kind of dog who is worth admiring and worth
ng - and that is what you want your dog to be! Here are
me of the things that you could teach him.

Spinning Around

Do this trick only when you know that your dog is ready as it
may make him dizzy. However, it is also fun to watch every once
in a while so that you could teach him this, too!

•   To let your dog go on a circular motion, use your touch stick
as a guide.

•   Now, when you see that your dog has gone into a circular
motion, use the clicker and reward him.

•   Lessen the use of the touch stick gradually and repeat the
process until the dog learns how to spin without the stick.

Jump through Hoops

You have probably seen this trick in the circus or most dog
shows. Well, you can teach this to your dog, too! All you have to
do is:

•   Place the hoop on the floor first then ask someone to hold it.
Ask your dog to come to the hoop.

• Repeat the said process until such time that your dog already feels comfortable going around the hoop.

• When that happens, you can now hold the hoop higher and then give a command by saying the word "leap" so your dog would jump through it. Do not forget to call him by his name, as well.

• Raise the hoop higher and ask your dog to leap then do not forget to use the clicker and give him a treat when he does.

Roll Over

This trick is one of the most popular dog tricks out there, and if you can help your dog learn how to do it then, by all means, you are on to something! To teach him this trick, just follow the instructions below.

• First, ask your dog to lie down on the floor.

• Then, use the training stick to guide him to where you want him to roll over. It is important that you see him use his back to roll. When he does this, use the clicker and reward him. Give a command by saying the word "Roll Over" so he will be able to connect these words with the trick.

• Repeat the process until he rolls over completely then stop making use of the training stick.

• When he rolls over without the stick, praise and pets him and don't forget to offer him a treat. Always make use of the clicker, too.

X Marks the Spot

Teach your dog to go to a place where you have marked with either an item or a marker. Here is what you have to do:

• First, wait for your dog to touch your training stick then give him a treat and use the clicker after.

• Then, place an item or a packaging tape on the floor as a marker then points towards it with the use of your training stick.

• Lead your dog to the spot by saying the name of the marker and when he comes to it, use the clicker and reward him.

• Repeat the process until your dog understands it.

Shake It Off

Before you sing that Taylor Swift song, take note that this is basically about teaching your dog how to shake. This is a fun trick and here is how you can teach him to do it:

• When he shakes his body after bathing, especially if he does not shake it off too much on you, use the clicker and reward him with a treat.

• Now, if he does it again, even if you have not bathed him yet or when he is completely dry, use the clicker and offer a treat once more. This will help him understand that it is okay to shake.

• Give a command by saying the word "Shake" and maybe move your body in the same manner, too. Offer a treat and use the clicker if he follows you.

That was fun, wasn't it? Practice these tricks and see how much more happiness your dog could bring you!

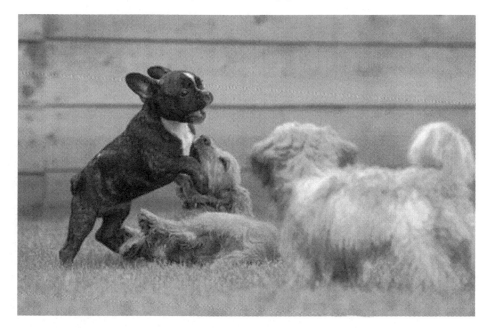

Chapter 12: Secrets of Living in Harmony with your Dog

Open a Door

Wouldn't it be cool if your dog knows how to close and open a door? For this trick, you need a towel or a bandana that you can tie on the knob so your dog can have something to tug on.

• Call your dog by his name and make hand signals that will help him realize that he has to tug on the towel that is hanging on the knob.

• Wait for him to do so and just be patient. Once he tugs on it and the door is closed, say "open" and wait until he tugs hard enough and the door opens. Use the clicker and give him a treat once he does the trick successfully.

• Repeat doing this until he learns to open the door by tugging.

Let us Count!

And finally, for the last day of training, it would be nice if you could teach your dog how to count. It is one of the best tricks out there, and it will impress a lot of people! Here is what you have to do:

• First, sit across from your dog so you would be able to face each other.

• Hold your right hand up and hold a treat with your other hand then look at your dog in the eye. This will prompt him to bark.

• Once he barks, reward him with a treat. Ensure that you repeat the process for him to bark another time then drop your hand. Reward him once he does.

• **Repeat the process until he understands that he will receive a reward if he barks until you put your hand down.**

Hush, Hush

Some people say that one of the main reasons why dogs make good pets is the fact that dogs bark at strangers. However, sometimes, they could be a little too territorial, and they may also bark at people you want them to be friends with such as your friends or some of your relatives. And of course, that would be a bit annoying because you really wouldn't like to spend your time asking your dog to stop barking, would you? Well, you can try to quiet him down by following the instructions below:

• Look at your dog while he barks unnecessarily then wait for him to stop. Or, call him by his name and say "Stop" and wait until he does so.

• Once he does, use the clicker and offer a treat.

• Now, give a command by saying the word "hush" to get him to quiet down and reward him with a treat.

• Repeat until necessary. You can also make use of hand signals so that your dog will be able to follow you easily.

Fetch

Now, this is one of those things that you usually see dog owners teach their pets. It is fun, and it makes for good playtime! Here is what you have to do:

• Ask your dog to pick something up on the floor and ask him to come to you so he could give it to you.

• Then, once the toy is in your hands, toss it away from him, but make sure that it is not too far that he cannot easily get to it.

• Tell your dog to pick it up and wait for him to do so then use the clicker and give him a treat once he hands it over to you.

• Do not worry about repetition. Dogs usually love this trick!

Jump Rope

If your dog knows how to jump, he should also learn how to jump rope! This is also a good form of exercise, so it is beneficial for your dog. Here is how you can teach him to do it:

• First, prepare a table that your dog could step on then tell him to "jump" on the table. Make sure that the table is sturdy so your dog will be safe.

• Use the clicker once he jumps and rewards him with a treat.

• Then hold the jump rope with one hand and tie the other end of it to another sturdy item, such as a pole then let the jump rope move back and forth, so your dog will realize how easy it is to move on it.

• Turn the jump rope, but stop once it comes across the legs of your dog. Give a command by saying the word "jump".

- When you see your dog jumping, slide the jump rope underneath him and use the clicker then give him a treat.

- Practice until he no longer has a hard time jumping on the rope!

Keeping his Toys

Dogs are like kids in the sense that they love to play. And that's why you also have to teach them to be responsible using keeping their toys in the storage if they are not using them. Here is what you have to do:

- Place a basket on the floor right next to you then put his toys on the floor.

- Ask him to pick up a toy, come to you, and "drop" the toy in the basket.

- Repeat until all of the toys on the floor are in the basket, then use the clicker and give him a treat.

- Say "Put your toys away" before asking him to pick up his toys, come to you, and drop the said toys in the basket.

- Repeat as necessary.

Chapter 13: Other Important House Training Tips

Now that you already have your basic plan, it's time to further reinforce the lesson with a few effective tips that can really help the process.

1. Prepare a den for him. As we've already mentioned, dogs in general are instinctively den animals. Most pups don't really want to spoil the area around them. But if you give them too much space, then they may want to relieve themselves in some nearby rooms. You can then gradually increase the space he can roam in your home. But at night, use a crate or a pen.

2. Don't let him see you clean up after his accidents. This should be done more privately. When you clean up after him after he does his business where he shouldn't, he may think that it's alright to do it there. It may seem to him that you approve, and he'll keep on doing it. Instead, take him to another room while you clean up.

3. Remove the scent from the accident area. Of course, you want to do this because the odor isn't all that appealing. But the main reason here is that your puppy tends to go to areas where his scent is strong and concentrated. So you should use a mixture of equal parts of vinegar and water to eliminate the scent. You can also use some alternative odor removal products from your local pet store.

4. Be careful about correcting bad behavior. Sometimes this works, and sometimes it doesn't. You have to know the difference.

For example, when your pup is about to does his business in an area where he isn't supposed to, you can startle him by making loud noises such as clapping your hands as you say "stop". You can even jump excitedly to get his attention and interrupt him. Once that's done, you should return to a more relaxed demeanor. You can calmly direct him to the right place. Then when he resumes his business, you can lather praise on him.

But this is perhaps the only possible use of "correction". Frightening him for something that he's done won't work. If he has an accident, you need to control your anger and frustration. He's not out to make your life miserable. It's simply part of your duty as a dog owner, which is pretty much like being a full-time parent.

5. Be careful about how you feed him. Puppies have special dietary needs, and you should be consistent about the brand of dog food you use. In fact, you should only choose a brand other than what he's used to if and when your vet suggests it. Puppies also tend to gorge, so you need to limit his food during feeding time. You don't just lay out food for him for all hours of the day either.

6. Watch for the food treats. Using food treats is always an effective training method, but it can affect elimination schedules. You may want to try a different motivational tool if your puppy keeps on doing his business at very random times.

7. Mind the water consumption. You should limit his intake of water too. But you have to watch out that you don't dehydrate your dog. Give him water when he's feeling extra lethargic or he's panting. You should prepare half a cup of water three times a day, and you can also consult your vet. But in general, you should stop offering your dog water by 7:30 PM or so, so that there are no accidents during the night when he sleeps.

Chapter 14: Dog Treating

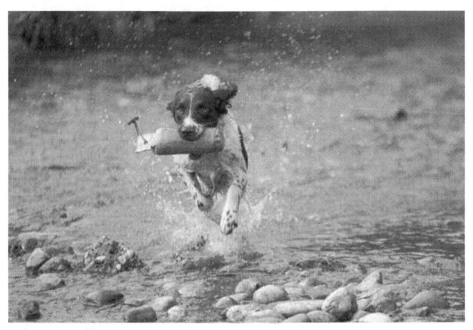

Treats, treats, TREATS! Come and get me'. How many times have you heard a friend or family member tell you about some crazy food that their dog loves? Dogs do love a massive variety of foods; unfortunately, not all of the foods that they think they want to eat are good or great for them. Dog treating is not rocket science but does take a little research, common sense, and paying attention to how your dog reacts after wolfing down a treat.

I am going to throw out some treats for training as well as some regular ole "Good Dog" treats for your sidekick and friend in mischief. I will touch on the proper time to treat, giving the treat, types, and bribery vs. reward.

Types of Treats

Love and attention are considered a reward, treat as positive reinforcement, and can be just as effective as an edible treat. Dog treating is comprised of edibles, praise, love and attention, as well as play or allowing some quality time with their favorite piece of rawhide. At times, these treats are crucial to dog training.

Human foods safe for dogs such as fruit and veggies, cut up meats that are raw or cooked, yogurt, peanut butter, kibble, and anything you come up with that your pup loves, but is good for him and his digestive system are all great for dog treating. Not all human foods are great for dog treating though, please read up regarding human foods that are safe for dogs.

Giving the Treat

Try to avoid treating your dog when he is over stimulated and running amuck and in an unfocused state of mind. This can be a counterproductive treating as it may reinforce a negative behavior or you may be unable to get your dog's attention.

When giving the treat allow your dog to get a big ole doggie whiff of that tasty food treat, but keep it up and away from a quick snatch and grab. Due to their keen sense of smell, they will know long before you figure it out that there is a tasty snack nearby. Issue your command and wait for him to obey before issuing the doggie reward. Remember when dog treating to be patient and loving, but do not give the treat until he obeys. Try to use the treating to reward the **kickback** mellow dog not the out of control or over-excited dog.

Some dogs have a natural gentleness to them and always take from your hand gently, other dogs need some guidance regarding taking the treat from your hand in a manner that is gentle. If your dog is a bit rough on the ole treat grabbing hand, go ahead and train the command "Gentle" when giving treats. Be firm that from this point forth no treats will be given unless taken gently. Being steadfast with this decision will work well and soon your pup or dog will comply if he wants his tasty treat.

Time to Treat

The best time to be issuing dog treats is in between his or her meals. If training always keep the tastiest treat in reserve in case you need to reel your dog's attention back to the training session. Too close to meal times all treats are less effective so keep that in mind when planning you training sessions. Obviously if your dog is full from mealtime he will be less likely to want a treat reward than if he is a bit hungry, therefore your training session is apt to be more difficult and far less effective.

What's In the Treats?

Take a gander at the treat ingredients and makes sure there are no chemicals, fillers, additives, colors and things that just seem unhealthy. Certain human foods that are tasty to us do not go down the doggie palette too well so take note. Almost all dogs love some type of raw meat and or slightly cooked meats. In tiny nibble sizes, they work great to get their attention where you want it focused.

Many people like to make homemade treats and that is fine, just keep to the rules we just mentioned and watch and read what you are adding while you are having fun in the kitchen.

Remember to read the list of vegetables dogs can and cannot eat, and note that pits and seeds cause dog's issues such as choking and intestinal issues such as gas. Remove the seeds and pits, and clean all fruits and veggies before slicing into doggie size treats.

Bribery vs. Reward Dog Treating

The other day a friend of mine mentioned bribery for action when he wanted his dog to shake his hand. I thought about it later and thought I would clarify. **Bribery** is offering the food in advance to get the dog to act out the command or behavior. **Reward** is giving your dog his favorite toy, food, love, affection after he has performed the behavior.

Example of bribery - you want your dog to come and you hold out in front of you a huge mound of steak in your hand before calling him. Reward would be giving your dog the steak after he obeyed the "Come" command and came to you.

Bribed dogs learn to comply with your wishes only when they see food, the rewarded dog realizes that he only gets his reward after performing the desired action. This is also good as other non-food items can more easily be introduced as rewards when dog treating.

Chapter 15: Dog Nutrition

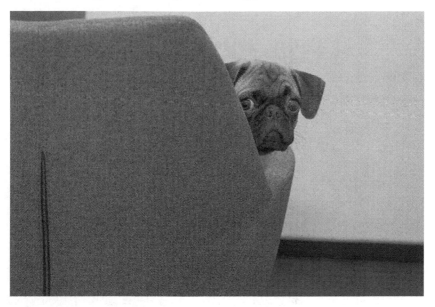

Nutrition, humans' study it, practice it, complain about it, but usually give into the science of it. The same as humans, dogs have their own nutrition charts to follow, different theories, scientific studies and so forth.

Together, let's look at history, common sense, raw foods, nutrient lists, and what your dog might have to bark about regarding what he is ingesting and thinks he can and cannot eat.

In the beginning there were wild packs of dogs everywhere, and what did they eat anything that they could? Similar to human's survival; dogs depended upon meat from kills, grasses, berries, and other edibles that nature provides. Guess what the great news is? Many millennia later nature is still providing all that we need.

Some History

In Roman history, the Romans wrote about feeding their dogs barley bread soaked in milk along with bones of dead sheep. The wealthy Europeans of the 1800's would feed their dogs better food than most humans had to eat. Dead horsemeat was oft rounded up from the streets to recycle as dog food to the rich estates on the outskirts of the city. Royalty is legendary for pampering their dogs with all sorts of delicacies from around their countries and elsewhere. Meanwhile, the poor's dogs had to fend for themselves or starve. Being fed table scraps from a pauper's diet was not sufficient to keep a dog healthy, and the humans themselves often had their own nutrition problems. Dogs would hunt rats, rabbits, mice, and any other rodent type creature they could sink their teeth.

Other references from the 18th century tell of how in France the French would mix bread crumbs with tiny piece of meat, or mix the liver, heart, blood, or all, with milk or cheese along with bread for feeding dogs. In England, they would also offer meat flavored soups to their canines to add to their dog's nutrition.

In the mid to late 1800's a middle class blossomed out of the industrial revolution. They started taking on dogs as house pets and created the enterprise of feeding the household pets that were suddenly in abundance. This new class with its burgeoning wealth had extra money to spend. Noting that the sailor's biscuits kept well for long periods James Spratt began selling his own recipe of hard biscuit for dogs in London, and soon after took his fare to New York City. It is believed that he started the American dog food business. This places the dog food and kibble industry at only a bit over 150 years old, and now is a multi-billion dollar business

All the while we know that any farm dog, or for that matter, any dog that can kill something and eat it will do just that. Nothing has changed throughout the centuries. Raw meat does not kill dogs, so it is safe to say with some common sense and diligence a raw foods diet will not either.

Raw Food Stuff

Let us take a look-see at the raw food diet for canines. First remember our dogs, pals, best friend, comedy actors, were meant to eat real foods such as meats, either cooked or uncooked. Their DNA is not formed only to eat dry cereals concocted by men in white lab coats. These cereal and canned foods may have been keeping our pets alive, but possibly not thriving at optimum levels.

There are many arguments for the benefits of real and raw foods. Sure it is more work, but isn't their health worth it? It is normal, not abnormal to be feeding your dog, a living food diet; it is thought that it will really boost their immune system and over-all health. **All foods** contain a risk, dry, wet, or raw they can all contain contaminants or parasites.

There are different types of raw food diets. There are raw meats that you can prepare at home, freeze-dried, and frozen that you can easily thaw and feed your dog.

Raw food diets are foods that are not cooked or sent through a processing plant. Only you can decide what you think is the type of diet for your dog, but it is worth the research effort to read up on a raw foods diet or mix of kibble and raw foods.

Rules of thumb to follow for a raw food diet

1. Before switching make sure your dog has a healthy GI track.

2. Be smart and do not leave meat un-refrigerated for lengthy periods.

3. To be safe simply follow human protocol for food safety. Toss the smelly, or does not seem right meats and foods.

4. Keep it balanced. Correct amount of vitamins and minerals, fiber, antioxidants, and fatty acids. Note medical issues and correlation.

5. Gradual switch over is often recommended to let their GI track adjust. Use new foods as a treat then watch stools to see how the dog is adjusting.

6. Take note of the size and type of bones thrown to your dog. Not all dogs do well with real raw bones.

7. Freezing meats for three days, similar to sushi, can help kill unwanted pathogens.

8. Take notes about what is working and not working with your dog's systems. Remember to be diligent in observation and note taking to track new diet.

9. Like us humans, most dogs do well with different foods. There is no one size fits all diet.

10. Please read up on raw foods before switching over, and follow veterinary guidelines.

Chapter 16: The Beginning of a Good Routine

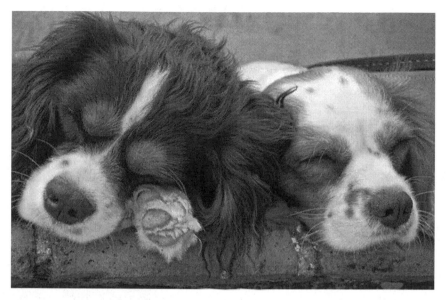

Puppies are cute and oh so cuddly. It is extremely easy to pamper them and this will turn them into brats when they grow up. Things that puppies do might seem endearing when they are young. However, the same things might become annoying when they grow up. Therefore, it is extremely important to get your puppy used to a routine.

Morning

As soon as your pup gets up in the morning, you should take him outside to do his business. You can make use of verbal cues like "hurry hurry" or "go do potty." You can make use of treats and praises for rewarding him when he does his business outside. This will definitely encourage him to keep up this behavior. Make sure that you are taking your puppy for a walk only after he has done his business. If the puppy is two months old, don't walk the pup for more than ten minutes. This helps in ensuring the pup's bones and joints are growing well and without any added strain. Once you are done with the walk, it's time for the pup to have his breakfast. After breakfast, take the pup for a walk again. Before leaving to work, you should take the puppy for a walk again.

Afternoon

Puppies are capable of holding their bladders for up to one hour per month of their age. If you work from home, then you can take your pup out in the afternoon. However, if you work away from home, then you will need to make necessary arrangements. The pup will need to be taken out for a walk at least twice in the afternoon as well. If you keep your pup in a crate and the crate is away from the door, then carry your pup out during the first few weeks. You will have to give your puppy lunch in the afternoon. Pups need to eat at least three times a day until they are six months old and then twice a day. Consult your veterinarian for the suitable feeding schedule.

Evening

This is the best time for you to bond with and train your puppy. As soon as you get home, take your puppy out of the crate and take him for a walk. Let your puppy do his business. Take your puppy out for a while. Take him to a park, a sports field or anywhere where he will get to meet and interact with different people. He will need to explore and get used to a variety of surroundings. Avoid places where there might be too many dogs until your puppy has had all his 16-week vaccinations. Encourage your pup to interact with other healthy dogs. Spend time with the pup in the evening and teach him a few good manners and commands. Teach your puppy basic commands like sit, heel, down, come and drop. Make sure that each session isn't more than 10 minutes since the attention span of a puppy is quite short. Make use of his kibble or treats for rewarding him.

Bedtime

The last thing that you will need to do before you go off to bed would be to take your puppy out for doing potty. Whether your puppy gets to sleep in his crate or with you is your call. If your puppy is sleeping beside you, then make sure that you close the door or that you are using a baby gate. Puppies are quite curious and you don't want him going off alone into the night to explore. The results are often undesirable. Puppy-proof your house. In fact, this should have been done prior to puppy arriving!

Water and Housebreaking

You will need to provide your puppy with fresh and clean drinking water while you are housetraining him. Your puppy needs to get a cup of water per 8 pounds of his body weight. Controlling your puppy's water intake would mean that you can control his output as well. However, restricting the amount of water might make your pup drink too much when he does have access to water. Give your puppy half a cup of water at least 20 minutes before you put him in his crate. Don't give your puppy any water an hour prior to his bedtime. Your puppy will need to go out for potty as soon as he wakes up, after he plays, after eating and drinking, and also after every 10 minutes of being taken out of his crate.

Chapter 17: Guideline on Puppy training

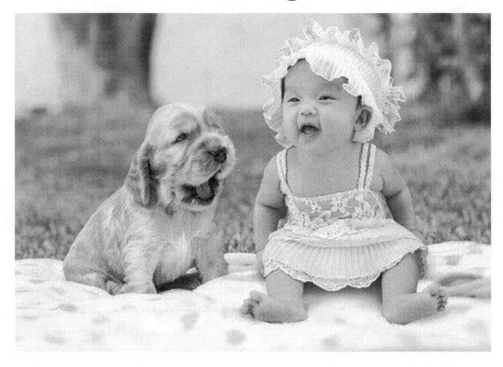

Reward

As you are implementing the steps above, practicing repetition, being consistent, establishing a routine and setting attainable goals, it is time to focus on rewards. It is human nature to work on a reward system. People perform actions because there is a pay-off in the end. That doesn't mean all actions are done with selfish motives as sometimes the payoff is that the actions make another person feel good. But rest assured there is always a pay-off, be it a warm fuzzy feeling, a paycheck, staying out of trouble or some form of gratification or relief.

Dogs function on the same level. They work for a pay-off in the end. It is easiest to begin with the payoff being in the form of something they can see, taste and chew. Give your dog his reward treat immediately upon completion of the task but do make sure it is not given until the task is completely finished successfully.

Especially if you are doing a good bit of regular training, be sure that the treats you are giving are healthy ones. Read the labels. Some of the most popular brands are the worst for your pet. It is worth spending the extra money to ensure that you are giving your dog treats that aren't laden with bad ingredients and are healthy for him, instead. You can limit the size of the treats by buying smaller ones or breaking off pieces of larger sized ones.

In addition to giving treats, it is a good idea to bask him with love and affection. Praise him and let him know you are pleased and proud. This goes a long, long way with a dog whose very ancestor domestication evolvement stemmed around working for and being needed by humans. It is in his genes to want to please. In fact, it is believed that years and years ago, dogs adapted to being useful as workers and as a means of survival. In return for work or for being helpful, they were rewarded with food, shelter and generally, affection as well. The instinct to please people is still in most dogs. Learn to tap into that trait and use it in your training sessions and you will go far.

After your dog has caught on to the trick at hand, wean him from the treats as the sole means of reward. If you don't wish to continue using treat rewards, that is fine. Even if you do plan to continue rewarding with treats, though, it is still best that you follow this step every now and then to get him away from the mindset that there must be a treat in front of him in order to perform the task. That thinking can be dangerous if you are in an emergency situation where he needs to obey immediately and there is no time to grab a treat.

When you are weaning him off the treat system, do so gradually. Every other accomplished trick or task gets a treat and every other warrant a shower of affection. Advance to every third time gets a treat with two rounds of affection in between. Be sure the affection turns are hearty and that they last at least 20-25 seconds.

As your dog matures with the concept of learning, you can lessen the energy behind the affection and the length of time of it as well. Just as a parent praises a child for learning a task like riding a bike or learning to count, eventually the amount of recognition dwindles and it becomes something that is just done and not acknowledged each and every time the activity is performed. The slight difference is that you will want to acknowledge your dog each time but it can certainly graduate to a minimum.

Tone

As the trainer, you are in charge. You set the tone, which is the overall mood of the sessions. Your tone will greatly determine how your dog feels about the lessons in general. Your calm and cool, assertive demeanor will help him to enjoy the lessons rather than dread them.

Don't think you can easily pull one over your dog. They are quite attuned with nature and with how their master is feeling, physically and emotionally. If you are having trouble getting into the proper mode, take some time to wind down. Meditate, take a run, talk to a good friend or read a book to get you distressed and focused on the session.

Keep the tone of your training times consistent. You don't want to be up one time and down another, in a good mood one day and a bad mood the next. Such variations will only confuse and upset your dog. Keep the mood the same each time so your dog knows what to expect.

It is a good idea not to be too energetic and excited when training your dog because you can easily excite him and make it difficult for him to pay attention and focus on the lesson. At the same time, being too serious and mundane is not a good idea, either. Keep your tone right in the middle and the two of you will do fine.

Positivity

Everyone responds better when positivity abounds. Children learn better in positive situations and with teachers who point out good things rather than bad. It is a proven fact that bosses who treat their employees with affirmations have much better workers. Dogs react very well to positive strokes, too.

Be sure to keep your sessions positive. Each and every trick or command you give should be done so in a positive manner. Rewards or corrections should be done in a similar way. It is not enough, though, to only be positive in training. You must also carry that into everyday activities so your dog does not ever fear getting on your bad side or upsetting you. If he does, he will be paranoid and worried during sessions which will be a huge distraction.

A positive atmosphere promotes fun and when your dog is having fun, he is automatically going to be on the same page as you. The two of you will be in tuned without even trying because, it just takes over. Consider Colby Jack who lives in the mountains of Colorado. He takes his dog everywhere in a dog-loving village where he lives. The two have a great rapport and an unbreakable bond so it is only natural that his dog, Dakota, follows his instructions when asked to "slide". Dakota goes up the short stairs all by herself and slides down the slide, time after time. She loves it because he and Colby are having fun. And if you think that is too complicated and advanced for you and your dog, you might reconsider. "It was incredibly easy to train Dakota because she loves to have fun and loves to please me," says Colby. Colby is just thirteen years old.

When you think of training your dog as fun and enjoyable, your dog will believe the same. Dogs are very intuitive. Not only are you teaching your dog new things, you are preparing him to be a great citizen who will be well received. The two of you are spending quality time together and are getting a chance to bond. You are blessed to have your dog and in return, your dog is blessed to have you. What is there not to love about the honor of training your pooch? Make it positive because...it IS positive!

Positivity is contagious. When you keep your sessions optimistic, you are confident in your dog's ability to learn and that will spill on over to the way he thinks. He will pick up on your attitude and most likely adopt it for himself. As the saying goes, if you think you can, then you really can. So give your dog the positivity he deserves.

The Perfect Pro to Train Your Dog

When it comes to training your dog, there is a pro that is highly recommended. YOU! You are the dog's master. You are the one he is with the most and whom he is most attached to, so it makes sense that you are the perfect match when it comes to be his trainer. With the tips and techniques lined out in the easy steps within this book, you will be able to be as professional as any other trainer you might seek out.

"Anyone can be trained to train their dog," states Gena Zaby who has been training dogs for more than thirty years. "You must become one accord with the animal you are training and the rest is a piece of cake. Knowing your dog and your dog knowing you are great bonuses you have to your advantage but I can meet any dog and immediately begin to train him and with the tools you can learn in dog training books like this one, you can do the same."

Dog training for dummies is an approach for those who know little about dogs and even less about training. Even if you fall into this category, there is something that can teach you so you can master the task and gives you clues on the secrets of dog training even if you feel less than qualified. Following the easy steps in this dog training book is a practically fool-proof way to train a dog like a pro, even if you are far from being one.

There is nothing wrong with having someone else train your dog, like a licensed trainer and there are situations that warrant such like an aggressive dog or one who is up for getting licensed to give assistance. But in general, since you will be the one with your dog and the one who will be giving him the commands or requesting him to do the tricks, it is optimal that you be the right one to teach him. And besides, the bond between a dog and his master will enrich the relationship that binds the two of them together.

Chapter 18: Dealing with Separation Anxiety

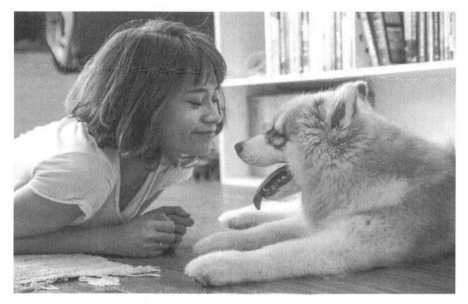

Puppies hate being left alone. If it is up to them, they will probably follow you to the end of the World. But, they cannot. As much as you both enjoy your time together, there are times when you simply have to leave your pooch alone, and chances are, you have to do it on a daily basis. But just because you hear sad whining when you close the door doesn't mean that your pup is anxious you left them alone. In order for you to be able to help them cope better with separation, you will first need to determine whether it really is anxious or not.

So, what are the signs of separation anxiety in puppies? If your pup is chewing things destructively when left alone, keeps urinating and defecating even if it is house trained, is barking, howling, and whining excessively, develops a habit of excessive digging or keeps scratching the door as an attempt to reunite with you, chances are, your pooch is suffering from separation anxiety.

Do not despair! This is completely normal, and it happens in the majority of cases when the dog owner has a full-time job that requires them to leave the house for longer periods of time.

Here are some tips that can help you knock down the anxiety and boost the mood of your pooch a bit while you are away:

-        Do not make departures and arrivals a big deal. Keep ignoring your pup while getting ready to leave the house, and then gently pet them on the head before you leave the door. Do not turn to mush with them only to show them your back and close the door. Leaving with kisses and treats will not reassure your pooch. Quite the contrary. That will only leave them stressed out.

-        Come up with a "Goodbye" word that you will use every time you leave your home. That will reassure your pup that you will actually get back.

-        Make sure to leave the area where the pup will be staying dimly lit, so you can encourage sleep.

-        Always leave toys around. Giving your pup something to chew on while alone is a great way for them to keep boredom at bay and not think about being left alone that much.

-        If needed, leave the radio on playing relaxing music such as classical music or jazz, if you need to cover unfamiliar sounds and offer reassurance. The best advice is to play that music even when you are together in the house so that your pup will get used to it.

-       Spend some time near their crate so that their safe haven will smell like you even after you leave the house. Some owners even leave recently worn pieces of clothes around so that the area will still have a strong scent of you.

-       If you come home only to find a mess, do not yell or correct your pup. The correction will not be associated with the destruction that the puppy has caused, but with your arrival. Instead of teaching them to be more disciplined in the future, you are actually contributing to them feeling even more anxious the next time you leave the house. Instead of correcting, try to find a different approach to ensure that the destructive behavior will not happen again.

-       If your pup is suffering from severe separation anxiety, consult with your veterinarian. They may suggest you hire a dog walker to take them on long walks, or even for you to sign your puppy up for a doggie daycare.

Keep in mind that separation anxiety is not a result of lack of training. This form of anxiety and obedience have nothing in common, so don't fool yourself into thinking that insufficient training is what causes your pooch to behave destructively when you leave the door. Follow the tips above and see if you can offer reassurance. If you keep providing reassurance from the early stages, your pup will soon learn to accept the routine and you will have no problem to leave your full-grown dog alone when going out in the future. Give it some time and be patient.

Conclusion

For many people, pets are just a great part of life. A part of life that can be hard to train sometimes. There are lots of tips on adult dog training available these days, and I would like to talk about a few of them.

While many pet owners have adult dogs that have never been trained before, many owners realize that having a well-trained pet in the house is much easier on them.

There are many ways that you could train your dog, depending on what you want to accomplish with him. If you want him to do complex tricks that will obviously take a lot of time, and you will want more detailed help.

If you simply want your dog not to go potty in the house or become accustomed to a crate, that is very doable in a short amount of time.

Obedience training is a great way to introduce your dog to be happy, non-anxious and behaved, to correct behavior problems in adult or younger dogs. There are traditional methods, such as classical conditioning available for you if you are looking to correct some simple behavior problems like social anxiety.

When classical conditioning is used, the animal will be introduced to a situation that he does not like very much. The reason for this is that it will make him get accustomed to those situations. Before long, the anxiety and fear of those situations can completely vanish for him.

One very popular tip for training your dog is to use kibble or some treat to lure him into doing simple commands. This is called a lure-reward and can be very effective for both puppies and adult dogs.

I hope this book was able to help you to know how to teach your dog some tricks!

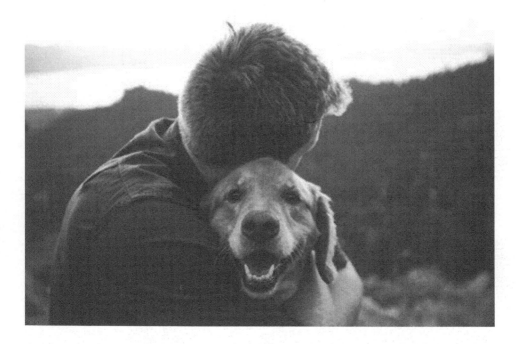

Dear dog lover,

If you enjoyed this book, don't miss the second volume!

Dog Training Basics: The Beginner's Guide to Raising the Perfect Dog with Positive Dog Training. Includes Puppy Training, Crate Training and Potty Training for Puppy

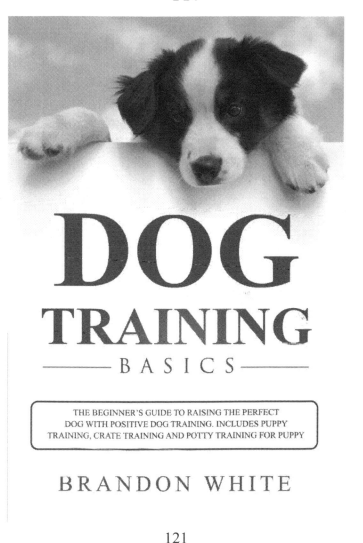

DOG TRAINING — BASICS —

THE BEGINNER'S GUIDE TO RAISING THE PERFECT DOG WITH POSITIVE DOG TRAINING. INCLUDES PUPPY TRAINING, CRATE TRAINING AND POTTY TRAINING FOR PUPPY

BRANDON WHITE

Made in the USA
Lexington, KY
15 November 2019

57057768R00068